THE SOVEREIGN PATIENT

HOW AI EMPOWERS PATIENTS AND CAREGIVERS TO TAKE CONTROL OF THEIR HEALTHCARE

DAN NOYES

The Sovereign Patient

Copyright © 2026 by Dan Noyes

All rights reserved. No part of this book may be reproduced in any form or by any electronic or mechanical means, including information storage and retrieval systems, without permission in writing from the publisher, except by reviewers, who may quote brief passages in a review.

ISBN: 979-8-9941871-4-2

Medical Disclaimer

This book is designed to provide information and guidance about navigating healthcare systems and understanding medical AI. It is sold with the understanding that the author and publisher are not engaged in rendering medical, health, or any other kind of personal professional services in this book.

The information in this book is based on the author's personal experiences, research, and opinions. It should not be considered a substitute for professional medical advice, diagnosis, or treatment. Always seek the advice of your physician or other qualified health provider with any questions you may have regarding a medical condition. Never disregard professional medical advice or delay seeking it because of something you have read in this book.

The author and publisher specifically disclaim all responsibility for any liability, loss, or risk, personal or otherwise, which is incurred as a consequence, directly or indirectly, of the use and application of any of the contents of this book.

If you have or suspect you have a medical problem, promptly contact your healthcare provider.

AI and Technology Disclaimer

The discussions of artificial intelligence, medical technologies, and healthcare systems in this book reflect the state of these rapidly evolving fields as of the publication date. Technology capabilities, regulations, and healthcare practices may change significantly over time. The author and publisher make no representations about the accuracy or completeness of information regarding specific AI tools, medical devices, or healthcare technologies mentioned in this book.

Readers should verify current information about any medical technology or AI tool with qualified healthcare professionals before making healthcare decisions.

Published by Sovereign Health Press

Printed in the United States of America First Edition: 2026

DEDICATION

To Julie - For seeing the sovereign in me when I could only see the patient. Your belief gave me the strength and support to lead my journey, and your love made sure I never walked it alone.

DEDICATION

HOW TO USE THIS BOOK

This book is organized into sixteen chapters, but you don't have to read it cover to cover. Living with a chronic condition means your energy is precious. Some days you have the bandwidth for deep reading. Other days you need a quick answer to a specific problem. This guide is designed to work either way.

If you're reading straight through, the chapters build on each other. The first section (Chapters 1–5) explains what's broken in healthcare and how AI is already shaping your care. The middle section (Chapters 6–9) gives you practical tools: how to evaluate AI, ask better questions, coordinate your team, and protect your data. The final section (Chapters 10–16) goes deeper—defining your values, transforming your conversations with providers, planning for the future, and honoring the emotional reality of chronic illness.

But if you need something specific right now, start here:

If you have a doctor's appointment this week → Start with Chapter 7 (Asking Better Questions) and the Question Preparation Card inside it. Then read Chapter 11 (The Conversation That Transforms Care) for communication strategies that work.

If you're overwhelmed by managing your condition → Start with Chapter 12 (Your Patient Action Plan) for the Health Dashboard and 30-Day Challenge. These frameworks can bring order to the chaos.

If you're curious about AI in healthcare → Chapters 3 (The Invisible Algorithms), 4 (Finding My Second Brain), and 6 (What AI Can and Can't See) will give you a clear-eyed view of what AI does well, where it falls short, and how to use it wisely.

If you're worried about your health data and privacy → Chapter 5 (Your Right to Understand) covers informed consent and what you're actually agreeing to, and Chapter 9 (Your Data, Your Rules) gives you practical steps to protect your information.

If you're struggling emotionally → Go straight to Chapter 16 (The Feeling Nobody Prepares You For). It's the conversation nobody has with you about grief, exhaustion, isolation, and self-compassion. You may also want the Three AM Practice and Self-Compassion Reset at the end of that chapter.

If you're a caregiver → Chapter 8 (Orchestrating Your Healthcare Team) addresses the unique challenges of coordinating care for someone you love. Chapter 10 (Defining What Matters to You) will help you have the values conversation that makes everything else clearer.

If you're newly diagnosed → Read Chapters 1 and 2 first. They'll help you understand why the system feels the way it does—and that it's not your fault. Then skip to Chapter 10 to start defining what matters to you before the system defines it for you.

Every chapter ends with tools you can use immediately. You'll find Question Cards, template scripts for difficult conversations, decision-making frameworks, and practical protocols throughout. Think of this book as a reference guide you can return to whenever you face a new healthcare challenge. Dog-ear the pages. Highlight the scripts. Keep it next to your medical binder.

Most importantly, there is no wrong way to read this book. Start wherever you need to start. Skip what doesn't apply right now. Come back to the rest when you're ready. Sovereignty isn't about doing everything perfectly. It's about taking whatever step you can, whenever you can.

1

———

WHEN HEALTHCARE STOPPED SEEING YOU

The fluorescent lights hummed with potential as I watched my new neurologist's face. His eyes darted between me and the screen, where my medical history glowed in neatly organized tabs. This was my fourth neurologist.

I had prepared meticulously for this appointment. I'd been journaling symptoms, tracking medication effects, documenting the seemingly random patterns of my seizures. I had even created a visual timeline linking traumatic brain injuries to the cascading neurological symptoms that followed. I arrived with printed charts, carefully organized notes, a folder thick with documentation.

But as I sat in the cold examining room, I realized none of that preparation mattered. The doctor wasn't reading my carefully crafted narrative. He was scrolling through drop-down menus, clicking through standardized forms, navigating a digital architecture that had no place for the wisdom I'd earned through suffering.

"You're a very unusual case," he finally said, eyes still fixed on the screen where my life had been reduced to diagnostic codes and test results. "You don't fit any of the standard protocols. In fact, you're one of the most challenging patients I've seen."

I had heard those words before. Challenging patient. The medical euphemism for inconvenient. For difficult. For someone whose experience refuses to be contained in checkbox fields and standardized workflows.

Then something unexpected happened.

His gaze finally met mine. Something shifted in that moment of genuine connection, a flicker of understanding that transcended the algorithmic expectations separating us. He set aside the keyboard.

"Tell me what it's like," he said. "Not the symptoms. What it's like to live with this condition day to day."

My throat tightened. When was the last time a doctor had asked me that question? When had anyone in the healthcare system wanted to know about my lived reality rather than their internal quantifiable metrics?

I described the cognitive fog that descended without warning, stealing my words mid-sentence. The bone-deep fatigue that felt like wearing a lead blanket. The seizures that left me disoriented and frightened, sometimes in public places where strangers became unwitting witnesses to my brain's betrayals. The shame of losing my consulting business because clients couldn't rely on me anymore. The grief of watching my identity dissolve with each new symptom.

As I spoke, I watched him listening, truly listening, not just waiting to translate my words into billable documentation. I realized what made this moment so rare: he was treating me not as a data source, but as a knowledge partner. Not as a statistical anomaly, but as a person with expertise about my own body.

"The system isn't built for patients like you," he admitted. "It's designed for predictable cases. When you don't fit the template, it gets clumsy. But people who don't fit the template often show you what matters most, in the body and in the system."

In that moment of clarity, I understood something fundamental about my experience navigating healthcare. The problem wasn't with my body. It came from a mindset that wanted to extract, not understand.

THE EXTRACTION PARADIGM

If you're reading this book, chances are you've felt it too. That sense of being invisible. Of bringing your whole self to a medical appointment, your fears, your observations, your hard-won understanding of your own body, only to have it distilled down to numbers on a screen that someone types while barely making eye contact.

You are not imagining it.

Modern healthcare has undergone a quiet transformation. It didn't happen overnight, and it wasn't announced in a memo. But over the past two decades, medicine has shifted from treating patients as whole persons to treating patients as data points. From valuing your story to extracting your information. From partnership to extraction.

I call this the extraction paradigm: medicine's quiet transformation of patients from partners to products, from storytellers to data sources.

The system isn't broken. It's operating exactly as designed, to optimize efficiency rather than empathy, to extract value from the very suffering it records.

Here's how it works:

When I describe my symptoms to a physician, a quiet conversion occurs. My lived experience, the fog, the fatigue, the fear, becomes alphanumeric. The cognitive difficulties become G93.3. The seizures become G40. Each code carries a reimbursement rate, an actuarial meaning, and a future bias embedded in algorithms I'll never see.

This isn't just paperwork. It reflects a belief system. It can make suffering profitable and make care feel transactional.

I didn't see it at first, until I realized that every code, every entry, was part of an invisible marketplace where my vulnerability had value. The data generated from my encounters would travel farther and last longer than the care itself.

Think about what happens after you leave the exam room. Your diagnosis becomes a billing code. That code can end up in insurance systems, where your future cost gets modeled. It feeds into pharmaceutical company analytics, helping them identify market opportunities for drugs you might need. It can shape how insurers and reviewers judge "medical necessity," which affects prior authorizations, what gets approved, and how hard you have to fight for the next step.

Your suffering becomes predictive data. Your vulnerability can start to feel like someone else's advantage, not what's best for you. We may not be able to prove it in every case, but many patients feel it.

A lot of the extraction is hard to see. You sign consent forms in legal language, and it's not always clear how your data will be shared. You may be told it's for "quality improvement" or "research" without understanding that these terms encompass commercial uses you'd never imagine. You might assume your data is protected by privacy laws, not realizing how many loopholes exist for "de-identified" information that can often be re-identified with surprising ease.

And here's the paradox: while your data is extracted, analyzed, and monetized with increasing sophistication, you often can't access that same data in formats you can actually use. Try getting your complete medical records in machine-readable formats. Try understanding what risk scores have been calculated about you. Try discovering which algorithms have made decisions about your care. The asymmetry reveals whose interests the system was designed to serve, and it wasn't yours.

The Research Behind Extraction

This isn't just my story. This pattern has been documented and studied, and many people believe it's getting worse.

Here's a shocking fact: For every hour your doctor spends talking to patients, they spend two more hours typing notes into the computer system. Think about that. One hour listening to you. Two hours typing about you.

And it gets worse. The average patient gets interrupted after just eleven seconds of speaking—a finding from a landmark study by Rhoades and colleagues published in the Journal of General Internal

Medicine. Eleven seconds. That's barely enough time to say "My back has been hurting and I'm worried because—" before your doctor cuts you off.

This isn't because your doctor is rude or doesn't care. It's because they're trying to do two things at once: listen to you and type everything into the computer. Their brain is split between the person sitting in front of them (you) and the screen demanding they fill in all the required boxes.

It's like trying to have a serious conversation with someone while they're texting. Even if they care about what you're saying, half their attention is somewhere else. They're going to miss things. They're going to interrupt. Not because they want to, but because the system makes it nearly impossible to do both well.

And here's what this does to doctors. When you're forced to treat people like data points instead of humans, it breaks you. Doctors didn't go to medical school because they love typing. They went because they wanted to help people. But the system makes them spend more time documenting than healing. That conflict wears them down.

And burned-out doctors make mistakes. When they're exhausted from hours of computer work after seeing patients all day, they miss things. They make errors. The more time the system forces them to spend on paperwork, the more dangerous it becomes for patients.

Think about what gets written down versus what gets ignored. Your doctor might spend thirty seconds asking about your symptoms. Then they spend ten minutes typing it all up in a way that satisfies the insurance company, the billing department, and the lawyers.

But here's what doesn't get documented: How scared you are. How this illness is affecting your ability to work or take care of your kids. What it feels like to live in your body right now. The pattern you've noticed that doesn't fit the textbook description. All of that—the human stuff, the stuff that actually matters to you—often disappears completely.

Not because your doctor doesn't care. But because the computer system has no box for "patient is terrified" or "this is ruining her life."

There's no billing code for listening to what matters most to you. And there's definitely no time for it when the next patient is already waiting.

This isn't just one problem here and there. This is the entire healthcare system changing its priorities. It used to focus on caring for people. Now it focuses on collecting data about people.

And you? You're experiencing this every time you sit in that exam room watching your doctor type while you're trying to explain what's wrong. You're living through it every time you get interrupted eleven seconds into talking. You're feeling it every time your doctor seems more focused on their computer screen than on your face.

This is what healthcare has become. And it's affecting your care whether you realize it or not.

How Did We Get Here?

It's easy to blame technology. To point at the electronic health record and say, "That's the problem." But the extraction paradigm predates modern computers. It began to shift when healthcare systems started measuring success by throughput instead of outcomes. By volume instead of value. By what could be counted instead of what counted.

Technology didn't create this problem. It accelerated it.

Meanwhile, physicians spend almost 4.5 hours daily on documentation and administrative tasks. Nearly two-thirds of doctors report spending more time with their electronic health record than with their patients.

These aren't just numbers. They reflect what people lose.

The loss of eye contact. The loss of story. The loss of what Francis Peabody meant when he said, "The secret of the care of the patient is in caring for the patient."

But here's what's crucial to understand: your doctor didn't choose this. The physician sitting across from you, typing while you talk, is as trapped by this system as you are. They went into medicine to heal, to connect, to serve. Not to become data entry clerks. Not to spend more time satisfying algorithmic requirements than understanding your lived reality.

So how did we get here? It didn't happen overnight. It happened through a bunch of government programs and insurance company rules that all seemed like good ideas at the time.

First, the government said all doctors had to use electronic medical records. Good idea, right? Paper charts were a mess. But the new computer systems were so complicated and demanded so much data entry that doctors ended up spending more time typing than treating.

Then insurance companies started paying doctors based on whether they checked certain boxes. Did you ask about smoking? Check. Did you record the patient's weight? Check. Did you document their blood pressure? Check. Sounds reasonable—until you realize doctors started focusing on filling out forms instead of actually listening to patients.

Then came a new payment system that was supposed to save money. Insurance companies started using computer programs to predict which patients would be expensive. High score? You're a "risky" patient. Low score? You're "low-risk." But real people don't fit into simple scores. Your life is complicated. Your health is complicated. The computer doesn't care.

Each rule made sense by itself. But when you stack them all together, you get a system where the most important part of a doctor's job became documenting data, not caring for people. The actual patient sitting in front of them? Almost an afterthought to getting all the boxes checked.

The Economics of Extraction

Want to know why this keeps happening? Follow the money. Your medical information isn't just being collected to help you. It's being sold.

Companies are buying and selling information about your health problems. Right now. Without asking you. Without telling you.

Here's how it works: Every time you see a doctor, get a prescription, or have a test done, that information goes into a database. Then companies buy lists of patients with specific conditions. "3.2 million people with diabetes." "850,000 people recently diagnosed with cancer." They package it up and sell it to whoever will pay for it.

Who's buying? Drug companies who want to target you with ads. Insurance companies looking for reasons to raise your rates or deny coverage. Marketing firms who want to sell you products. Anyone with a credit card and a "business reason" can buy information about your health.

You never said they could do this. Nobody asked your permission. But it's happening every single day, and it's completely legal.

This is why the system won't change. Your data is too valuable. The sicker you are, the more valuable your information becomes. Someone is making money every time a doctor types your diagnosis into that computer. And they're not about to give that up just because it's making your healthcare worse.

Your vulnerability has literal monetary value to entities you'll never interact with, who will use your health information in ways you'll never know. The patient with multiple chronic conditions isn't just expensive to treat, they're valuable to data brokers precisely because their complexity creates rich data profiles.

This isn't conspiracy theory. It's documented business practice. And it explains why the extraction paradigm is so entrenched: too many powerful interests profit from it. The system isn't failing to see you as a whole person. It has been designed to see you as a data source, because that's what generates value in the current healthcare economy.

Understanding this isn't meant to make you cynical. It's meant to make you informed. Because you can't change a system you don't understand, and you can't reclaim power you don't know has been taken.

What Doctors Are Losing Too

Before we go further, I want to be clear about something: this is not a book about doctor-blaming. Because physicians are casualties of the extraction paradigm too.

Dr. Abraham Verghese, a physician and professor at Stanford, coined the term "iPatient" to describe what happens in modern healthcare: the chart becomes more real to clinicians than the person in front of them. Not because doctors don't care, but because the system demands so much attention to the digital record that the actual patient fades into the background.

Verghese describes the phenomenon with painful clarity. He watches medical students and residents spend hours crafting detailed notes in the EHR, perfecting documentation, but spending mere minutes at the patient's bedside. The iPatient, the version that exists in the computer, gets meticulous attention. The real patient often gets a brief, distracted encounter.

Survey data reveals the depth of physician frustration: over 80% report that electronic health records interfere with their ability to provide quality care. The burnout epidemic among physicians, with nearly half reporting symptoms of emotional exhaustion and depersonalization, is directly linked to the loss of meaningful patient connection. Doctors went into medicine to heal people, not to feed data into systems that reduce human suffering to billing codes.

When your physician struggles to make eye contact, when they seem distracted by the screen, when they miss the emotional weight of what you're trying to say, it's not callousness. It's cognitive overload in a system designed to prioritize documentation over dialogue.

I've talked with physicians who describe a profound sense of moral injury, the pain of being forced to practice in ways that violate their core values. They know they're not giving patients the attention they deserve. They feel the disconnection. They grieve the loss of the doctor-patient relationship they trained for. But they're trapped in systems that measure productivity by patient volume and documentation completeness, not by the quality of human connection or the depth of therapeutic relationships.

This matters for your journey toward sovereignty. Your physician isn't your adversary. They're often trapped in the same extractive system. When you advocate for yourself, when you push for partnership, you're not fighting your doctor. You're fighting alongside them against a paradigm that serves neither of you.

The path forward requires recognizing that physicians and patients share a common enemy: a healthcare system that has lost sight of care itself.

The Journey to Invisibility

My own path to understanding this began on a winter afternoon in upstate New York. I was on the roof of our home, clearing snow, when the ladder shifted beneath me. The world tilted. Then came the impact, shoulder first, then my head.

My wife drove me to the emergency room, where physicians treated the shoulder fracture but missed the traumatic brain injury. No concussion protocol. No cognitive assessment. No follow-up plan. Just a fracture to be coded, billed, and closed.

I left with my arm in a sling, my brain silently damaged, and my future forever altered by what had been overlooked.

In the months that followed, I developed increasingly severe neurological symptoms: seizures that felt like moments stolen from time, and episodes where consciousness simply vanished.

During one family vacation in Phoenix, I lost awareness while driving. When I "came back," I had no idea where I was, who I was, or why I was behind the wheel. The terror of that moment, the realization that my brain could betray me without warning, changed everything.

What followed was a cascade of specialists, medications, and consultations, none of which captured the totality of my experience. One neurologist prescribed medication at twenty times the recommended amount. That overdose nearly ended my life.

What followed was months of hospitalization and rehabilitation, relearning basic functions the medication overdose had stolen: how to read, to write, to speak coherently.

My business collapsed while I was unable to work. My identity, my livelihood, and my autonomy, all casualties of a system that reduced me to data points while missing what mattered.

Eventually, I became my own archivist. I documented every seizure, every trigger, every environmental factor that preceded them. I arrived at appointments with charts and graphs, determined to bring my experience into the clinical conversation.

One doctor refused to even look at my notes.

The message was clear: patient-generated knowledge didn't count.

That's when I began to understand that invisibility isn't just a side effect of illness, it is a design feature of the extraction economy.

Looking back now, I can see the precise moment I crossed from being a person receiving healthcare to becoming a subject of extraction. It wasn't during the fall. It wasn't even during the missed diagnosis. It was in that neurologist's office, watching him refuse to acknowledge the hundreds of hours I'd spent learning my own body's language.

The emotional impact of that dismissal was profound. It wasn't just frustration, it was a fundamental destabilization of my sense of self-worth. If my most careful observations didn't matter, if my lived expertise counted for nothing, then what value did I bring to my own care? The system was teaching me that I was irrelevant to my own healing.

I began to second-guess everything. Were my symptoms real or was I imagining patterns that didn't exist? Was I being a demanding patient, expecting too much from overworked physicians? Should I just accept whatever treatment was prescribed and stop asking questions?

But something else was happening too. As I connected with other patients navigating chronic illness, in online communities, in hospital waiting rooms, in rehabilitation facilities, I began to recognize my experience everywhere. Different conditions, different bodies, different circumstances, but the same essential erasure. The same reduction to data. The same dismissal of patient knowledge.

Think of Sarah, a member of an online diabetes community. She's 32 years old, carefully managing Type 2 diabetes while working full time and raising two kids. She came to an appointment with Dr. Cara Webster with detailed food logs, blood sugar readings meticulously tracked over three months, and a pattern she'd noticed: her glucose spiked every Friday morning, even when she ate the same breakfast as other days.

"I think there's something about my work week stress that affects my blood sugar," Sarah explained, showing Dr. Webster her carefully organized data. "I don't see it in the textbook, but the pattern is consistent."

Dr. Webster glanced at the logs and smiled, but Sarah noticed something shift. The doctor's eyes went to her computer. A few clicks. A quick review of the lab results glowing on screen.

"Your A1C is where we want it," Dr. Webster said. "Keep doing what you're doing with your diet and exercise. The stress observation is interesting, but I'd focus on what the numbers tell us."

Sarah left feeling both validated and erased. Her diabetes was well-controlled. But the insight she'd earned through three months of careful observation, the knowledge she'd developed about her own body, had been politely dismissed in favor of a single lab value.

She is not alone in this experience. Many patients bring detailed observations to their appointments, only to have those insights treated as anecdotal noise rather than data worth investigating. The extraction system runs in one direction: from patient to record. Patient-generated knowledge, no matter how carefully gathered, doesn't flow back in.

Julie is a 42-year-old single mother of two teenagers, managing chronic pain from a car accident five years ago. The accident left her with nerve damage that doctors describe differently depending on which specialist she's seeing. Some call it fibromyalgia. Others say it's a nerve condition. One suggested it might be autoimmune.

What Julie knows is this: on most days, her body aches in ways that make simple tasks feel monumental. Getting out of bed takes strategy. Playing with her kids is done in carefully rationed doses. Work is manageable only because she can rest between meetings.

She saw Dr. Leo Park, a new physician at Riverside Hospital, hoping for fresh perspective. Before the appointment, Julie noticed something: the risk algorithm on the clinic's system had flagged her as "high utilizer" due to her multiple visits over the past year. The algorithm didn't capture why she'd been coming frequently. It just noted volume.

"You've been here quite a bit," Dr. Park mentioned, eyes still on the screen. "We want to make sure we're not just managing symptoms. Have you considered that some of this might be psychological?"

Julie had considered it. She'd tried therapy, mindfulness, cognitive behavioral approaches. These things helped, but they didn't make the pain disappear. She hadn't come to the appointment expecting that they would.

But sitting there, hearing her utilization pattern reframed as potentially psychosomatic, Julie felt something familiar: the system's quiet message that her complex, chronic reality was somehow a failure of her mental fortitude rather than a legitimate medical condition. The algorithm had made a judgment, and the physician was channeling it.

These are just two examples of how the extraction paradigm compounds already difficult experiences. The system takes your data, analyzes it through algorithmic lenses, and returns interpretations shaped by what the system can measure and code, not by what you actually live.

You Are Not Alone

Perhaps you recognize yourself in these stories. Maybe not the specific details, your condition is different, your symptoms are different, your journey is uniquely your own. But the feeling? The frustration of being unseen? The experience of bringing your full complexity to a medical encounter only to have it reduced to boxes on a form?

That feeling is universal among patients navigating modern healthcare.

You might be the patient with chronic pain whose descriptions are dismissed because they don't match what the algorithm predicts. The mother whose intuition about her child is overridden by a risk score. The person of color whose symptoms are interpreted through biased lenses embedded in medical AI. The elderly patient navigating digital systems designed for a different generation. The person managing multiple chronic conditions whose complexity breaks every standardized protocol.

The details vary, but the extraction feels the same.

Enter Artificial Intelligence

Now, artificial intelligence is transforming healthcare at a pace most patients don't fully grasp. Algorithms are making decisions about your care, decisions you might never know about. They determine how long you wait in the emergency room. And in 2026 whether your insurance approves a surgery. Which treatments get recommended. How your risk is calculated.

The integration of AI into healthcare is happening largely without patient awareness or input. You might not know that an algorithm helped determine your hospital discharge date, or influenced whether you were flagged for a follow-up call, or calculated a fall risk score that shaped your nursing care plan. These decisions happen in the background, shaping your care in ways you never see.

The invisibility is built into the process. AI systems in healthcare are often described in vague terms, "clinical decision support or CDS," "workflow optimization," "quality improvement tools," language that obscures their actual role in shaping your care. You're rarely told when an algorithm has influenced a decision about you, let alone given the opportunity to question its logic or challenge its conclusions. This asymmetry of information creates an asymmetry of power.

And the pace of AI adoption is accelerating. What took decades to unfold with electronic health records, the gradual shift from partnership to extraction, could happen with AI in a matter of years. The question isn't whether AI will transform healthcare. It's whether that transformation will serve patients or further extract from them.

I experienced this firsthand during a recent visit. My physician suddenly moved away from traditional note-taking to a new ambient AI scribe that captured every word in a much more conversational way. The system promised to ease documentation burden, and it did. My doctor could finally maintain eye contact. We could actually have a conversation.

But I also learned something unsettling: the software wasn't just transcribing. It was analyzing paralinguistic cues to assess patient "reliability" and "compliance probability." It was recording my tone, my pauses, even my hesitations.

I remember wondering: could it read my unease? Could it register the silence between my answers? And what would happen to those assessments?

Mary is a 58-year-old marketing manager. She's also a caregiver. Her mother has early-stage Alzheimer's, and Mary spends two hours every morning helping her with basic tasks before heading to work.

She came to see Dr. Susan Chang one afternoon, exhausted and anxious. "I'm not sleeping well. I'm worried all the time. I don't know how much longer I can manage both my job and my mother's care," Mary said. It came out in a rush, the weight of two years of caregiving suddenly visible in her voice.

Dr. Chang listened, then turned to her computer. Mary watched as the physician's fingers flew across the keyboard, entering codes: caregiver stress, anxiety, sleep disturbance. On the screen, these became billable diagnoses.

"I'd like to start you on something for anxiety," Dr. Chang offered. "And I can refer you to our social worker for caregiver resources."

Both suggestions were helpful. But Mary left the appointment feeling like something crucial had been missed. She didn't need a diagnosis. She needed to be heard. She needed someone to understand that her anxiety was rational, given her circumstances. She needed acknowledgment that what she was carrying was unsustainable, and that the solution wasn't to medicate her reality away but to help her navigate it.

The system had converted her lived experience into codes and treatment recommendations. It had diagnosed her rather than understood her. And in doing so, it had made her invisible as the whole person she is: a woman trying to balance impossible demands, a daughter honoring her commitment to her mother, a professional maintaining her responsibilities, all while losing sleep and losing hope that anyone in the healthcare system truly grasped what she was carrying.

What Mary needed wasn't extraction of her symptoms into a list of diagnoses. The system demanded the coding, but Mary needed partnership. Partnership in figuring out what "health" could realistically look like for her in this season of life. Partnership in understanding not just what she's carrying, but why, and what might genuinely ease her burden.

These are the invisible costs of the extraction paradigm. Not just the loss of dignity or the feeling of being unseen. But the fundamental mismatch between what patients need and what systems are designed to provide.

This is what makes invisible algorithmic decision-making so urgent. It operates at scale, at speed, and often without transparency. A biased human clinician can harm patients one at a time. A biased algorithm can harm thousands before anyone notices the pattern.

Research increasingly documents how AI triage systems, risk prediction tools, and clinical decision support algorithms carry embedded biases. A 2024 study in Nature Medicine found that several widely used triage algorithms were systematically deprioritizing patients from certain zip codes, not because of medical necessity, but because the algorithms had learned from historical data that included structural biases in how those patients were treated.

Think about what that means. The algorithm wasn't creating a fairer system. It was automating and scaling existing inequities.

This is the promise and peril of AI in healthcare. Used well, it could free doctors to focus on patients. It could catch patterns humans miss. It could amplify patient voices instead of silencing them.

Used poorly, it becomes surveillance medicine, the transformation of care into continuous data capture, where every word, every pause, every expression feeds algorithms you'll never see or understand.

So here we stand at a crossroads. AI could entrench the extraction paradigm, making it faster, more efficient, more inescapable. Or it could become a tool for liberation, helping patients reclaim their voice, their knowledge, and their rightful place as partners in their own care.

The difference between those futures hinges on one question: Who decides how AI is used in your healthcare?

The Path Forward

This book is about reclaiming your role in that decision. It's about moving from subject to sovereign, from passive recipient of algorithmic decisions to active partner in AI-augmented care.

Over the following chapters, I'm going to share what I've learned, not just from my own journey through medical complexity, but from working at the intersection of healthcare and technology, from studying how systems can serve or subjugate patients, and from the growing community of people who refuse to accept invisibility.

You'll learn:

- How to recognize when AI is being used in your care (it's happening more than you think).
- The questions that reveal hidden algorithmic bias and force transparency.

- Why your knowledge about your own body is as important as any algorithm's predictions.
- How to document and present your experience in ways healthcare providers will take seriously.
- What partnership with your healthcare team actually looks like in the age of AI.
- Practical tools to advocate for yourself without alienating the people trying to help you.
- How to help create a healthcare future where AI serves patients instead of extracting from them.

This is not a book about rejecting technology or fighting with your doctors. It's about understanding the systems shaping your care so you can work with healthcare providers to ensure AI amplifies your voice rather than silencing it.

Because here's the truth: you have more power than you think. And the healthcare system needs you to claim it.

What Sovereignty Means

The word "sovereign" might feel like a big word for a patient book. But I use it deliberately.

A sovereign is not a subject. A sovereign has agency, the right to understand, to question, to participate in decisions affecting their life. A sovereign is not ruled by invisible forces they cannot see or comprehend.

In healthcare, sovereignty means:

- You have the right to know when algorithms are making decisions about your care.
- You have the right to understand how those algorithms work and what they're considering.
- You have the right to question algorithmic recommendations.

- You have the right to contribute your own knowledge and experience to clinical decisions.
- You have the right to define what health and flourishing mean for YOUR life.

These aren't radical demands. They're basic requirements for informed consent in an age where consent often happens without patients even knowing algorithms are involved.

Claiming sovereignty doesn't make you difficult or demanding. It makes you an informed participant in your own care. And that benefits everyone, including your healthcare team.

A Note on Hope

I need to be honest with you: this book is born from frustration and pain. From lying on a bathroom floor, confused and bleeding. From watching my identity dissolve under the weight of medical complexity. From the soul-crushing experience of being told my carefully documented observations didn't count as "real" data.

But it's also born from hope.

Because I've also experienced the opposite. I've sat across from clinicians who asked about my lived reality and truly listened. Who valued my observations as data worth considering. Who partnered with me to understand patterns the algorithms missed.

I've seen healthcare systems starting to include patients in AI governance. I've watched patient advocates ask questions that revealed algorithmic bias technical experts never thought to look for. I've witnessed the transformation that happens when patients are treated as knowledge partners instead of data sources.

The future I'm describing in this book isn't fantasy. It's already happening, just not everywhere. Some clinicians and patients are pushing back and building something better.

Our work is to weave these ideas into a clear vision you can use. I want sovereignty to be something you can expect, not something you have to fight for. And I want AI to be a tool that supports patients, not one more way they get processed.

And it starts with understanding. With recognition. With naming what's happened so we can begin to change it.

Your Story Matters

As you read this book, I want you to hold on to this: your experience is valid. Your knowledge about your own body is real. Your frustration with being unseen is justified.

You are not too complicated. You are not too demanding. You are not imagining the ways healthcare has stopped seeing you as a whole person.

The extraction paradigm is real, but you have more power to change it than you've been led to believe. You aren't just being difficult, despite how other may try to make you feel. I would often tell my wife, "My doctors aren't going to be sending me any Christmas cards, but that is ok. I'm here to take care of me, not to make friends. I will be nice and respectful, but I must be my own advocate."

Every chapter that follows is another step on medicine's journey from extraction to sovereignty. Some stretches will feel familiar; you'll recognize your own experience reflected back. Others may unsettle you with how much is happening behind the scenes. But I hope you'll stay with me.

Not because I have all the answers. I don't. But because we're learning this terrain together.

And together, we can reclaim what's been taken: your voice, your knowledge, your rightful place as a partner in your own care.

Welcome to the journey from subject to sovereign.

Your Turn: What Has Your Care Felt Like?

- Before moving to the next chapter, take a moment to
  reflect on your own experience. You might want to write

your thoughts in a journal or simply sit with these questions:

- When was the last time you felt truly seen by a healthcare provider?
- Have you ever brought observations or documentation to an appointment and felt they were dismissed?
- Can you recall a moment when you felt reduced to a data point rather than treated as a whole person?
- What would it mean for you to be treated as a knowledge partner in your own healthcare?
- What would change if you approached your next appointment as a sovereign rather than a subject?
- Hold onto your answers. They'll guide you through the rest of this journey.

2

───────

WHY MY DOCTOR ACTS
LIKE A TEENAGER

I get jealous when I see my doctor.

Not in a weird way. It's just that he spends all his time in front of a computer. Like a teenager scrolling through social media at the dinner table, except instead of TikTok, it's my medical record. And instead of dinner, it's my health.

Do I really have his attention? His eyes are glued to the screen. I get quick glances as he's talking to me, or more accurately, as he's talking at me while typing. I know I don't have his full attention. It's like trying to have a meaningful conversation with someone who's checking their phone every three seconds.

One time, I knew I had really lost him. His eyes hadn't left the screen in what felt like minutes. So I did something probably inappropriate: I glanced over at his computer screen.

He was Googling my symptoms.

I wish I could say I was exaggerating. Google. At least use Gemini, Claude, or ChatGPT, I thought. Give me some AI-powered search if you're going to phone it in.

But then something unexpected happened. As my initial frustration eased, I moved alongside him. I crossed the invisible line that separates patient territory from doctor territory in exam rooms. It felt like trespassing. He looked uneasy at first, like I was supposed to stay on my side of the room and him on his. Like I'd crossed some great chasm, this artificial divide we're supposed to maintain.

And then we started researching my issue together. I even shared with him how he might want to consider MedGemma, part of the Google family, if he wanted to do more in-depth research on my condition.

I was having terrible restless leg syndrome at night that was keeping me from sleeping. I wasn't sure if this might be connected to my chronic condition or if it was an interaction between drugs. I'm on seven different medications, because when you have complex health issues, you become a walking pharmacy, and I was wondering about cumulative effects.

I was actually shocked he could access Google from his computer in the examining room. Later, I learned he also had AI tools, but he had to sneak those on his personal phone because the medical system hadn't approved them yet. Think about that: a doctor smuggling AI into appointments like a teenager hiding their phone during class.

As I moved next to him, looking at the same screen, I explained my logic. Since all medications have pharmacological properties, chemical structures that interact with our bodies, was there potential that the chemical property of one was interacting with another or perhaps with several other drugs? Or could it be the cumulative effect of being on seven different medications for years, causing a problem that might have gone undiscovered because no one was looking at the whole picture?

He listened intently. Really listened. Then he said something that floored me: 'You know your condition and your medications better than I do.'

No ego. Just honesty. Honest collaboration. He agreed with my reasoning about the medication interaction. We made a plan together.

I was optimistic. This was what healthcare should feel like. Collaborative.

Then his time was up and he was on to the next patient.

One Month Later

My next visit was different.

Same doctor. Same exam room. But the magic was gone. He spent the entire visit updating my electronic health record. No eye contact. No collaboration. Just filling out forms about my visit. Click, click, type, type. The wall between us had gone back up.

He was tired. Exhausted, really. It showed in every movement, every word, every defeated slump of his shoulders.

So I asked him how he was feeling.

I can't make this stuff up. The patient asks the doctor if they're okay. But here's what I've learned: at the end of the day, doctor and patient are just two human beings trying to fulfill our purpose in life. I'm not a victim and he's not a savior. We're equals. Although he is far smarter than I would ever hope to be. This perspective might make me a better patient, or it might push me into the realm of being a 'difficult patient.' More about that later.

He looked at me like no patient had ever asked him that question. Maybe none had. Then his guard dropped.

'I'm overworked and exhausted,' he admitted. 'I spend up to four hours after seeing patients just to keep up. Reviewing electronic health records, refilling prescriptions, checking portal messages, ordering tests, reviewing results. The list goes on.'

Four hours. After a full day of seeing patients. I was beginning to wonder if he needed to see a good doctor.

'I didn't get into medicine to sit in front of a screen all day,' he said. 'But that's what's happening.'

That's when I started paying attention.

The Pattern Emerges

I began noticing it everywhere. Most of the time I have a medical visit, doctors and nurses spend most of their time at a computer. Not occasionally. Not sometimes. Almost always.

I volunteer at a local hospital, so I see this from multiple angles. Clinicians are seeing patients while simultaneously juggling data entry. Nurses updating records while checking vitals. Specialists are documenting while examining. The computer has become as essential to modern healthcare as the stethoscope.

The stethoscope draws them closer to your body, but sadly, the computer seems to be pulling them away from your story.

So how did this happen? How did we get to a place where doctors act like teenagers glued to their screens, not because they want to, but because the system requires it?

The History We Need to Understand

The thing is, electronic health records weren't created to torture doctors and annoy patients. They were created with genuinely good intentions.

Let me take you back to the not-so-distant past when medical records were entirely paper-based. Doctors scribbled notes by hand, often illegibly. Those notes stayed in file folders in one office. If you saw a specialist across town, they had no idea what your primary care doctor had found. If you ended up in an emergency room, they were working blind. Medication lists got lost. Test results never made it from the lab to your doctor's desk. Critical information lived in silos.

People died because of these gaps. They died from medication interactions that no one caught because no one had the full picture. They died from allergies that weren't communicated. They died from duplicate tests and missed diagnoses because crucial information was locked in a file cabinet somewhere else.

Electronic health records were supposed to solve these problems. And in many ways, they have.

When I show up at a new specialist's office, they hopefully can see my complete medication list. When I end up in an emergency room, which has happened more times than I'd like to count, they know my seizure history, my traumatic brain injury, my medication sensitivities. That information has probably saved my life. However, there is one important caveat: they all need to be able to talk together or data suddenly starts going missing.

Electronic health records can also catch things humans miss. They flag potential drug interactions. They remind doctors about preventive screenings. They track trends over time that might reveal patterns no single appointment would show. They coordinate care across multiple providers.

These are genuinely good things. We need electronic health records. No one with any sense is arguing to go back to paper files and illegible handwriting.

But....

The Unintended Consequences

What no one anticipated when they were designing these systems: the electronic health record wouldn't just document care. It would fundamentally reshape how care gets delivered.

Because electronic health records aren't just medical records. They're also:

- Billing systems. Every click generates a code that determines reimbursement.
- Legal documentation. If it's not documented, it didn't happen, at least not in court.
- Quality measurement tools. Algorithms assess whether your doctor is meeting performance standards.
- Insurance gatekeepers. Prior authorizations, formulary checks, coverage determinations.
- Data extraction systems. Feeding information to researchers, policymakers, and increasingly, AI algorithms.

So when your doctor is typing during your appointment, they're not just recording what you said. They're:

- Choosing billing codes that accurately reflect the visit complexity, while avoiding codes that might trigger an audit.
- Creating legal documentation that protects them if something goes wrong.
- Checking boxes required by quality metrics that determine their compensation.
- Navigating insurance requirements that might prevent you from getting the care they're recommending.
- Feeding data into systems they don't control and often don't fully understand.

All while trying to actually listen to you and figure out what's wrong and how to help.

Is it any wonder they seem distracted?

The Documentation That Got in the Way

Sarah's blood sugar numbers had been unpredictable lately, despite years of careful management. She scheduled a follow-up visit with Dr. Webster, her endocrinologist, hoping for some fresh insight.

The appointment started well. Dr. Webster asked good questions. Sarah explained her recent stresses, her changing work schedule, the fact that she'd been less active. It felt like a real conversation.

And then, about halfway through, Dr. Webster's attention shifted. She glanced at her watch, then pulled up something on the computer. Sarah watched as the doctor's fingers flew across the keyboard.

'I need to get this visit documented while I remember the details,' Dr. Webster explained apologetically. 'I have back-to-back appointments and if I don't do it now, I'll be here until 8 PM trying to catch up.'

Sarah understood. But she also felt the moment slip away. The careful clinical reasoning that had been happening, the collaborative thinking, had to pause so Dr. Webster could satisfy the documentation requirements that come before the actual care.

This is the cruel reality of modern healthcare: time spent documenting is time not spent with patients. However, the system demands both. Be with your patients. Document everything. Do both perfectly. Do both simultaneously. And when you can't, when you're forced to choose between the screen and the person, know that whichever you choose, you'll be failing someone.

The Hidden Cost of Alert Fatigue

But wait, you might be thinking. Aren't all those alerts and warnings supposed to help? Aren't they catching dangerous drug interactions and preventing medical errors?

In theory, yes. In practice, something else happens.

Modern EHR systems generate constant alerts. A doctor prescribes a medication, and the system flags a potential interaction. They order a test, and the system questions whether it's necessary. They document a diagnosis, and the system suggests alternative codes that might reimburse better.

Some of these alerts are critical. Life-saving, even. A severe drug allergy. A dangerous interaction between medications. A contraindication that could cause serious harm.

But most warnings aren't serious. Most are things like "This medication might cause a minor side effect in some people." Or "The average patient shouldn't take these two drugs together"—even though you're not average and your doctor knows they're fine for you specifically. Or "Don't forget to fill out Form 247-B"—which has nothing to do with keeping you safe and everything to do with paperwork.

It's like if your phone gave you a warning every single time you did anything slightly risky. "Are you sure you want to cross this street?" "That coffee is hot—it could burn you." "You're standing near stairs—be careful!" After the hundredth warning, you'd stop paying attention completely. Even when the warning said something important like "Your house is on fire."

The problem is that the critical alerts and the trivial ones look exactly the same. Same pop-up window. Same urgent formatting. Same required clicks to dismiss.

So doctors develop what researchers call 'alert fatigue.' They start overriding alerts automatically, clicking through warning screens without really reading them, because the vast majority, studies suggest between 49 and 96 percent, depending on the system, aren't relevant to the specific patient in front of them.

And then comes the alert that matters. The one that's actually catching a dangerous interaction. The one that could prevent serious harm. But it looks like all the others. It's buried in the noise.

A 2024 study in JAMA Internal Medicine found that alert fatigue directly contributes to medical errors. Doctors miss critical warnings because they're drowning in trivial ones. It's like the boy who cried wolf, except the wolf is real and the boy is an algorithm that won't stop crying.

The tragedy is that these systems were designed with the best intentions, to catch human errors, to prevent harm, to keep patients safe. But by generating too many alerts, they've created a new kind of danger: the inability to distinguish signal from noise until it's too late.

When the Metrics Don't Match the Patient

Julie's chronic pain had brought her back to Dr. Park's office. Some days it's manageable. Some days it makes everything harder. Even breathing can become difficult at times. The chronic pain is simply excruciating at times. When asked to score her pain from 1 to 10, she looks for a number 10 times worse.

Last year, she started seeing Dr. Leo Park at a pain management clinic. He listens. He asks about her life, not just her symptoms. He thinks carefully about treatment options and the impact they could have on her life. Traditional pain medications could impact not only her, but also her family. Dr. Park is exactly the kind of doctor you want when you're dealing with complex, long-term pain.

But then the clinic implemented a new 'efficiency optimization' system. It tracks how long doctors spend with each patient and compares it to departmental averages. The idea sounds reasonable: identify bottlenecks, improve patient flow, reduce wait times.

Except the algorithm doesn't account for complexity. A patient comes in with straightforward pain and a clear treatment plan. Average time: fifteen minutes. Julie comes in with chronic pain, a complicated medication history, questions about interactions, and concerns about dependence. She's anxious about new treatment options. This patient needs thirty minutes.

The algorithm sees both as 'pain management.' It sees Dr. Park spending more than double the average time. It flags him as inefficient.

Month after month, the metrics showed Dr. Park spending 'too long' with patients. Part of his compensation is based on these metrics. He began facing a choice: rush through complex cases like Julie's to meet the numbers, or continue providing the careful care he knew these patients needed and take the financial hit.

This is what researchers call 'metric-driven medicine,' care shaped not by clinical judgment but by what the measurement system rewards. Dr. Park didn't go to medical school to practice assembly-line medicine. The system is literally paying him to approach care with that mindset.

A 2024 study in the New England Journal of Medicine found that productivity metrics are increasingly driving physician behavior in ways that compromise patient care. Doctors are shortening visits not because patients need less time, but because algorithms penalize them for taking more time.

Dr. Park continues to take the time his patients need. But he's also thinking about what comes next, because it's hard to sustain a career when the system that employed you to heal is now punishing you for doing it thoughtfully.

When the Algorithm Overrides the Doctor

Here's something most patients don't realize: sometimes your doctor wants to prescribe a medication, order a test, or recommend a treatment and the computer simply won't let them.

These are called 'clinical decision support systems,' and like electronic health records themselves, they were created with good intentions. The idea is that the system helps doctors by suggesting evidence-based treatments, catching potential errors, and ensuring best practices.

But many of these systems have evolved from offering suggestions to imposing requirements. They're coded with what are called 'hard stops,' actions the doctor literally cannot take without extensive workarounds, and 'soft stops,' warnings that require multiple clicks and justifications to override.

Let me give you a real example because it happened to me. A doctor wants to prescribe a medication that's not on the insurance formulary, the approved list of drugs the insurance company will pay for. The medication is medically appropriate. It's the best choice for this particular patient and their situation. But it's not on the list.

The EHR won't let the prescription go through without a prior authorization. Fair enough, insurance companies have processes. But here's what that actually means:

The doctor has to stop seeing patients to call the insurance company. Wait on hold. Navigate phone trees. Get transferred between departments. Finally, reach someone who can accept the prior authorization request. Explain why the formulary medication won't work for this specific patient. Perhaps cite medical literature. Argue the case.

This process can take thirty minutes to two hours. For a single prescription.

Often, the insurance company denies the request anyway. Then comes the appeal process. More phone calls. More documentation. More time away from patients.

Many doctors, faced with this obstacle, simply prescribe the formulary medication instead. Not because it's the best choice, but because the system has made the better choice impossibly difficult.

If you have a chronic medical condition, you've probably experienced this process firsthand.

Doctors ignore these alerts almost all the time. Depending on the computer system, they click past anywhere from half to nearly all of the warnings they see. They know most of them don't matter.

But here's the absurd part: even when they ignore a warning, they have to explain why. Click the button. Type a justification. Document their reasoning. Over and over, hundreds of times a day.

So the computer is both blocking them from doing their job AND demanding they explain why they're trying to do their job anyway. It's like having someone stand in your way, and when you try to step around them, they make you fill out a form explaining why you needed to move.

The system slows everything down twice: once when it throws up the unnecessary warning, and again when it forces the doctor to document why they ignored it.

What's crazy about all this: These computer systems were supposed to help doctors make better decisions. Instead, they're stopping doctors from doing what they know is right.

The computer doesn't just make suggestions anymore. It blocks things. It says "no, you can't do that" even when the doctor knows that's exactly what you need.

So your doctor is stuck. On one side, they know what would help you. On the other side, the computer system won't let them do it. They can fight the system—spend twenty minutes clicking through override screens and typing justifications—or they can give up and do what the computer allows, even if it's not quite right for you.

Either way, you lose time with your doctor. And you might not get the care you actually need.

Why the Teenager Analogy Works

Think about why teenagers are glued to their phones. It's not because they don't care about the people around them. It's because their entire social world lives in that device. Their friends, their reputation, their sense of belonging, it's all mediated through that screen. Not engaging means being left out, missing important information, losing connection.

For doctors, the computer screen has become equally inescapable. Their ability to practice medicine, to get paid, to avoid lawsuits, to meet performance standards, it all flows through that screen. Not engaging means missing critical information, making documentation errors, failing quality metrics, or worse, harming patients by missing an alert.

The difference is that teenagers choose to be on their phones. Your doctor doesn't have a choice.

They're not acting like teenagers because they want to. They're acting like teenagers because the system requires them to. The screen isn't optional. It's mandatory.

Doctors Are Not the Enemy

I need to remind ourselves something extremely important: our doctors are as trapped by this system as we are.

You're frustrated because you're not being seen as a whole person. They're frustrated because they're not being allowed to practice medicine the way they were trained.

You feel reduced to data points. They feel reduced to data entry clerks.

You wish they'd look at you instead of the screen. They wish they could.

Let's also stop for a moment and remember: doctors are incredibly smart. They were the smartest people in your high school. They survived the hell of medical school and residency. They take continuing education courses every year to stay current on the latest advancements in healthcare. They never stop learning.

These are people who entered medicine because they wanted to heal, to serve, to grow intellectually, to make a difference. Nobody goes through the torture of medical training because they dream of clicking checkboxes all day.

What They're Really Facing

Think about what your doctor's day actually looks like.

They're seeing people at their worst. People in pain. People who are sick. People in a place they don't want to be. People looking for fixes to situations that have no easy fix.

Imagine doing that all day, every day.

Those same people may be angry with them for not fixing things faster. Angry about the high cost of healthcare, as if they set the prices. Angry about prescriptions that might not even be able to be filled because of insurance coverage. Prescriptions that might cause more side effects than the original problem they were trying to help with.

They have fifteen minutes to make you feel heard, to diagnose complex problems, to explain treatment options, to address your fears, and to document everything in a way that satisfies multiple competing systems.

Then they do it again. And again. Twenty to twenty-five times a day.

And then they go home and spend more time on the computer because the documentation couldn't be completed during those fifteen-minute windows.

This is simply not sustainable. And increasingly, doctors are realizing it. Burnout rates exceed fifty percent. Many are leaving medicine entirely. My primary care physician recently told me he's moving off to a slow, rural hospital in Wyoming. The smartest people in your high school are deciding the career they sacrificed everything for isn't worth the cost anymore.

The Research on Physician Burnout

When I talk about physician burnout, I'm not relying on anecdotes. The research paints a devastating picture.

The Mayo Clinic's 2024 study on physician well-being found that 54 percent of physicians report symptoms of burnout. That's more than half. And the numbers are getting worse, not better, with each passing year.

But here's what makes this crisis different from ordinary job stress: researchers are increasingly using the term 'moral injury' to describe what physicians are experiencing. The concept comes from military psychology. It describes what happens when you're forced to act in ways that violate your core sense of purpose and identity.

This isn't just making doctors tired. It's breaking them emotionally. Think about why someone becomes a doctor. They spend four years in medical school. Three to seven more years in residency, working brutal hours for terrible pay. They go into massive debt. They sacrifice their twenties and early thirties. Why? Because they want to help people. They want to heal. They want to make sick people better.

And then they get out into the real world and discover they spend one hour helping patients and two hours typing about it.

That's not just exhausting. That's soul-crushing. Imagine training your entire adult life to do something, going into $300,000 of debt to learn how to do it, and then being told you can only spend a third of your day actually doing it. The rest of the time? Paperwork. Forms. Clicking boxes. Justifying your decisions to a computer.

This is why doctors are quitting. This is why good, caring physicians are leaving medicine in their forties and fifties when they should be at the peak of their careers. Not because the work is too hard. But because the system won't let them do the work they trained their whole lives to do.

And it gets worse. The most experienced doctors—the ones who've been practicing for twenty or thirty years, the ones who've seen everything—are retiring early. Not because they're tired. Not because they want to retire. But because they can't stand what the job has become. We're losing the best doctors we have because the computer systems have made their work unbearable.

Even more alarming: one out of every three doctors is seriously thinking about quitting medicine completely. Not cutting back their hours. Not switching to a different specialty. Quitting. Done. Walking away from medicine forever.

Let that sink in.

Why? Because the system they're working in has nothing to do with the reasons they became doctors. They signed up to heal people. Instead, they're data entry clerks who occasionally get to see patients.

When a third of all doctors are thinking about quitting, that's not a few bad apples who can't handle the job. That's the system itself being fundamentally broken.

This is not a problem we can afford to ignore. When we lose physicians to burnout, we lose their expertise, their experience, their institutional knowledge. We lose the very people who could help us navigate an increasingly complex healthcare system. And we create a vicious cycle: fewer doctors means higher patient loads for those who remain, accelerating their burnout, driving more to leave.

This is a crisis, and the research confirms it. And it's a crisis that affects every single person who will ever need medical care, which is to say, all of us.

If you're thinking, I don't have the energy to worry about my doctor's burnout, you're not wrong. Patients shouldn't have to carry that. But understanding what's happening on the other side of the screen can help you protect yourself: it helps you tell the difference between a good clinician trapped by a bad system and someone who simply isn't showing up for you.

The First Thing You Can Do

Understanding all of this doesn't fix the system. But it does something powerful: it changes how you show up to your appointments.

Because here's what I've learned: the first thing patients can do is make their doctor feel appreciated and seen.

I know. You're the one who's sick. You're the one in pain. You're the one who waited weeks for this appointment. Why should you have to take care of your doctor's feelings?

Fair question. But here's the pragmatic answer: when you make them feel seen, they're more likely to make sure you're seen. It's not manipulation. It's recognizing shared humanity.

I make it a habit to ask my doctors and nurses if they're genuinely having a good day. These are some of the hardest workers in any profession. People can be difficult, myself included. So I do two things:

I thank them for their service. Because they truly are serving their patients. This is not just a job. It's a calling, even when the system makes them question why they answered that call.

You'd be surprised how quickly the guard can drop. How a simple question, 'How are you doing today?' can shift the entire dynamic. How acknowledging their humanity makes them more able to acknowledge yours.

This isn't about being nice for the sake of being nice. It's strategic empathy. When you recognize that you and your doctor are on the same side, both trapped by a system that values efficiency over humanity, you can start working together instead of working against each other.

The Power of Simple Recognition

Mary had been running on fumes. It's a constant balancing act between work, caregiving, managing her mother's medical appointments, and taking care of herself, which often gets pushed to the bottom of the list.

One afternoon, Mary had an appointment with Dr. Susan Chang at her primary care clinic. It was a 2 PM slot, the deadly afternoon when doctors are already running behind, already exhausted from the morning's patients, already dreading the evening's documentation.

When her name was called, Mary walked into the exam room carrying two things: her usual folder of medical questions and concerns, and a large coffee in a to-go cup for the doctor.

'I know you work hard and don't get breaks,' Mary said simply. 'Thought you could use this.'

Dr. Chang looked at the coffee cup like Mary had handed her a winning lottery ticket. Her eyes got bright. For a moment, she looked like she might actually cry.

'Thank you,' the doctor said quietly. 'You have no idea. This is the first time a patient has done that in months.'

The appointment that followed was different. Dr. Chang still had to use the computer. She had no choice about that. But she also made real eye contact. She asked follow-up questions. She listened when Mary mentioned feeling overwhelmed by caregiving responsibilities and started asking how that was affecting her stress levels and health.

This distinction mattered. Instead of rushing to the prescription pad, Dr. Chang spent time exploring what stress and exhaustion were actually doing to Mary's body.

Fifteen minutes turned into twenty-two. The doctor was running even more behind schedule now. But she didn't rush. And when Mary left, both of them were smiling.

Dr. Chang reflected later: 'First time anyone's acknowledged that I'm human in about three months. Usually, I'm just the person who isn't moving fast enough, who can't fix things immediately, who represents everything frustrating about healthcare. Mary reminded me why I do this.'

Research on physician well-being consistently shows that feeling valued and appreciated directly impacts the quality of care. It's not that doctors need their egos stroked. It's when you're functioning on empty, emotionally, physically, spiritually, that small acts of recognition can be the difference between shutting down and staying present. Between going through the motions and genuinely connecting.

Mary's coffee cost maybe five dollars. But its impact on her care, and probably on the care of every patient that doctor saw for the rest of the day, was immeasurable.

Partnership Within Constraints

Recognizing shared humanity is the foundation. But there are practical strategies you can use to create a genuine partnership with your doctor, even within the constraints of the current system.

First, bring a printed summary of your current medications, recent symptoms, and key questions. Come prepared. I know this seems old-fashioned in the digital age, but here's why it matters: it saves your doctor from having to hunt through multiple screens in the EHR to find information that should be at their fingertips. Did that save time? They can spend it actually talking with you instead of clicking through your record.

Second, when your doctor is typing or seems focused on the screen, try asking: 'What's the computer telling you to do?' This simple question accomplishes several things. It acknowledges the system's presence instead of pretending it doesn't exist. It surfaces when the doctor is being overruled or constrained by algorithms. And it opens the door to collaboration on how to work within or around those challenges.

I've used this question several times, and the responses are illuminating. 'It's flagging a potential drug interaction, but it's not actually relevant in your case because...' or 'Insurance requires prior authorization for this test, which means I need to...' Suddenly, you understand what's happening behind that screen. You're partners in navigating the bureaucracy, not adversaries separated by it. This can also help you see the world through your doctor's eyes.

Third, offer to wait while they complete the necessary documentation. Near the end of your appointment, you might say: 'I know you need to finish entering this information. I'm happy to wait quietly for a minute while you do that, and then I have one more question.' This gives them permission to focus on the screen without feeling like they're ignoring you. It acknowledges the reality of their work instead of pretending it doesn't exist.

Fourth, when appropriate, request shared-screen access. Not in an accusatory way, not 'what are you hiding?' but in a collaborative way. 'Would it help if I looked at the screen with you while we talk through this?' Sometimes the answer will be no, and that's fine. But sometimes, as with my doctor during my restless legs syndrome research, crossing that invisible line can transform the dynamic entirely, at least for that appointment.

Fifth, learn to distinguish between different types of silence. When your doctor is quiet while looking at the screen, they may be thinking through what they're seeing. Or they might be clicking through required fields that have nothing to do with your care. You can ask: 'Are you thinking, or is the computer demanding something?' This helps you understand whether to wait patiently or whether it's okay to continue the conversation.

Finally, learn when to accommodate the system and when to speak up. Respect time constraints. They're real, and they're often not your doctor's fault. Don't bring seventeen different questions and concerns to a fifteen-minute appointment. But also don't let the system's pressures prevent you from asking what truly matters. Be organized and succinct. If something is urgent, say so clearly. If you need more time to understand a diagnosis or treatment plan, state that need.

The goal isn't to become a pushover who accepts whatever crumbs of attention the system allows. The goal is to recognize that your doctor is working within the same broken system you are, and to find ways to partner with them despite those constraints.

When you approach appointments this way, something shifts. You're no longer a patient waiting to be fixed by a doctor. You're two people working together to navigate a system that serves neither of you particularly well. That partnership, fragile and constrained as it may be, is where real healthcare happens.

What This Changes

When I crossed that invisible line in the exam room and looked at the computer screen with my doctor, something shifted. We weren't patient and doctor anymore, separated by our roles. We were two people trying to solve a problem together.

That feeling of being on the same team? That sense of collaboration? That's what healthcare should feel like all the time.

But it won't happen if you're sitting on opposite sides of the room, with you viewing the doctor as the enemy and them viewing you as another demand on their impossible schedule.

Understanding why your doctor acts like a teenager glued to their screen doesn't excuse poor care. But it does help you identify when you're dealing with a good doctor trapped by a bad system versus a doctor who's genuinely not serving you well. That distinction matters.

And when you find a good doctor trapped by a bad system? That's someone worth fighting alongside, not against.

Because the truth is, you need each other. They have medical knowledge and clinical expertise. You have knowledge about your own body that no algorithm can capture. Together, you might be able to navigate a system that wasn't designed for either of you.

Looking Ahead

The next time you're sitting in an exam room and your doctor is typing while you're talking, take a breath. Remember that they're not choosing the screen over you. They're trying to serve two masters: the person in front of them and the system behind them.

Ask them how they're doing. Thank them for their service. Look for opportunities to collaborate instead of just receiving care.

And if you're really bold? Next time they're looking something up, move alongside them. Cross that invisible line, if appropriate. Look at the screen together.

You might be surprised what happens when you stop being

patient and doctor, separated by roles and screens and expectations, and become two people working together to solve a problem.

In the next chapter, we'll look at the hidden algorithms already making decisions about your care, often without you or your doctor even knowing. But for now, remember this: the person sitting across from you, typing while you talk, is not your enemy. They're your potential ally in a system that doesn't serve either of you well.

And that recognition? That's where change begins.

A Moment to Consider

- Before moving to the next chapter, reflect on these questions:
- When was the last time you saw your doctor as a person rather than just a role? What made that possible?
- Have you ever asked your healthcare provider how they're doing? If not, try it during your next appointment?
- Think about your last appointment. Can you identify which parts of your doctor's behavior were their choices versus requirements of the system? For example, ask them which times of day are busiest for them.
- What would change if you approached your next visit to see your doctor as a potential teammate rather than as someone who should fix you?
- If you could change one thing about how electronic health records work, what would it be?
- Write down your thoughts. They'll help you navigate the chapters ahead.

3

———

THE AI HIDDEN IN YOUR CARE

I was staring at my MRI report, and I might as well have been reading ancient Greek. This is the exact wording from the report:

"FLAIR/T2 signal are present within the subcortical white matter the bilateral frontal lobes. There is mild bilateral parietal volume loss. A cystic lesion is visualized within the right posterior fossa associated with the right hypoglossal canal. This likely represents a benign perineural cyst or other nonaggressive entity. A smaller similar lesion is visualized within the left hypoglossal canal."

What does that even mean? Is my brain shrinking? Should I be worried? Is this related to my traumatic brain injury, or is this something new? Am I going to die?

My next neurology appointment was three weeks away. I couldn't wait that long to understand what was happening in my own head.

So I did what a growing number of patients are doing: I copied the radiology report and pasted it into an AI tool.

"Please explain this MRI report in plain language," I typed.

Within seconds, I had something I could actually understand. The AI explained that the white matter changes were common in people with my history, that the volume loss was mild and not necessarily alarming, and that "no acute abnormality" was actually good news. It meant nothing urgent was happening right now.

I could breathe again.

When I finally saw my neurologist, I showed them the AI-translated version. They looked surprised, then intrigued. "This is pretty accurate," they said. "Did this help you understand what we're seeing?"

It had. Enormously. But it also revealed something important: AI is already deeply embedded in healthcare. I'm just not always aware of it.

And here's the thing: that AI translation tool? That was me choosing to use AI. That was visible, transparent, in my control.

Most of the AI making decisions about my healthcare? I never see it coming.

The Invisible Algorithms

What most patients don't realize: artificial intelligence is already making decisions about your care. Not in some distant future. Right now. Today.

When you check in at the emergency room, an algorithm helps determine how quickly you get seen. When your doctor orders a test, an algorithm decides whether your insurance will cover it. When you're admitted to the hospital, an algorithm calculates your risk of readmission. When you fill a prescription, an algorithm checks for drug interactions.

These systems are working in the background, invisible to most patients, making judgment calls about your health every single day.

And most of the time, nobody tells you they're there.

FIVE TYPES OF HIDDEN HEALTHCARE AI

To understand just how pervasive these invisible systems are, it helps to categorize the different types of AI you're likely encountering in your healthcare journey, often without knowing it.

1. **Triage and Prioritization Systems:** These algorithms decide how urgent your situation is and how quickly you should be seen. When you call a nurse hotline and answer questions about your symptoms, an algorithm is often scoring your responses to determine if you need emergency care, an urgent appointment, or can wait. In emergency rooms, triage systems now incorporate AI to assess which patients need immediate attention based on vital signs, symptoms, and risk factors.

2. **Insurance and Authorization Algorithms:** Before you receive care, AI systems are evaluating whether it's "medically necessary," whether you've met prerequisites, and whether your insurance will pay. These algorithms enforce step therapy requirements, determine if treatments are "experimental," and calculate coverage based on rigid criteria that may not account for your individual circumstances.

3. **Clinical Decision Support:** While your doctor is making treatment decisions, AI systems running in the background may be offering recommendations, flagging potential drug interactions, or suggesting diagnoses based on your symptoms and test results. Sometimes doctors see these alerts and recommendations; sometimes the AI influences decisions without the physician even recognizing it as algorithmic input.

4. **Risk Prediction Systems:** Hospitals use algorithms to predict which patients are at high risk for readmission, complications, or deterioration. These risk scores influence how closely you're monitored, how quickly you're discharged, and what follow-up care is recommended. A high risk score might get you extra attention; a low score might mean you're sent home sooner than you should be.

5. **Administrative Screening:** Beyond direct clinical care, AI systems screen for potential fraud, allocate scarce

resources like ICU beds or transplant organs, and identify patients who might benefit from disease management programs. These algorithms operate at the system level, making decisions about resource allocation that ultimately affect individual patient care.

The common thread? In most cases, patients have no idea these systems are shaping their care. The decisions happen behind the scenes, embedded in workflows that feel like business as usual.

The Research on Hidden Algorithms

If my experience and these examples feel anecdotal, the research confirms that invisible AI in healthcare is both widespread and poorly disclosed to patients.

Here's the reality: AI is already making decisions about your healthcare, whether you know it or not. It's triaging your emergency room visit, flagging abnormalities in your imaging, recommending treatments, deciding whether you need a specialist referral. In most major hospitals today, AI influences most clinical decisions in some way. Yet most patients have no idea it's happening. The algorithm works invisibly, behind the screen, shaping your care without your knowledge or consent. You're already living in an AI-powered health-care system. The question isn't whether you'll encounter it. The question is whether you'll understand what's happening when you do.

AI algorithms are woven throughout your entire healthcare expe-rience. They're deciding when you get an appointment based on whether the system thinks you'll actually show up. They're flagging your account for collections before you've even missed a payment. They're recommending treatments based on what worked for other people, not necessarily what's right for you. And here's the kicker: the system almost never tells you any of this is happening. The algo-rithms are there, quietly making decisions, and you're expected to trust a process you can't see and didn't know existed.

And then there's insurance. This is where invisible AI gets truly dangerous. Insurance companies are using algorithms to deny claims at rates that would shock you. These aren't denials from doctors reviewing your case and making medical judgments. These are computers saying "no" based on coded criteria, with minimal human oversight. When you appeal a denial, you're not arguing with a medical professional who disagrees with your doctor. You're arguing with an algorithm that was programmed to reject a certain percentage of claims. Most patients never realize this. They think there's a person on the other end making a reasoned decision about their care. There isn't.

The FDA is smartly approving AI-enabled medical devices, from diagnostic imaging tools to surgical planning systems. Most operate invisibly to patients. When your mammogram is read, you probably don't know if AI pre-screened the images. When your dermatologist examines a suspicious mole, you likely don't know if an algorithm suggested it looked concerning. The technology is there, influencing clinical decisions, but disclosure is inconsistent at best.

This isn't to say all hidden AI is problematic. Many of these systems provide genuine value, catching errors, identifying patterns, improving efficiency. But the lack of transparency means patients can't distinguish between helpful AI and harmful AI. We can't consent to or question what we don't know exists.

When an Algorithm Decided How Long Sarah Waited

The following vignette illustrates how invisible algorithms can lead to dangerous delays in care.

Sarah was managing. That's the word she kept using—managing her diabetes, managing her stress, managing her schedule. One afternoon at work, she felt a tightness in her chest. Not crushing pain, nothing like she'd expected a heart attack to feel like. Just a persistent pressure, shortness of breath, and a cold sweat.

She drove herself to the ER, assuming it was probably stress or anxiety. The triage desk asked the standard questions: symptoms, history, risk factors. Sarah mentioned the chest discomfort, but when they asked about heart disease in her family, she said no. She was relatively young, no history of smoking. The triage algorithm, which uses AI to assess urgency based on symptoms and risk factors, categorized her as lower priority. After all, the algorithm reasoned, heart attacks are less common in women her age without a family history.

She waited three hours.

By the time she was finally seen by Dr. Marla Jones in the ER, she'd had a mild heart attack. It turned out that women often present with different heart attack symptoms than men, and the training data the system learned from was heavily skewed toward male patients. The algorithm had missed something crucial: women in their 30s can have heart attacks, and their presentation might look nothing like the textbook male presentation the AI was trained to recognize.

Sarah survived. But she had no idea an algorithm had influenced how long she waited. She thought it was just a busy night in the ER. The system had made an invisible decision about her care, and nobody explained that to her.

This is the reality of AI in modern healthcare: it's everywhere in its influence, and nowhere in its visibility to patients.

The Racial Equity Problem

Sarah's experience with gender bias in triage algorithms reveals a broader problem: AI systems often encode and amplify existing healthcare inequities.

Algorithms learn from historical data. And if that historical data reflects biased medical practices, the AI will replicate and sometimes magnify those biases. This isn't theoretical. It's documented, measurable, and causing real harm.

For decades, kidney function calculations included a race-based adjustment that assumed Black patients naturally had higher muscle mass and therefore different kidney function than white patients. This algorithmic adjustment, embedded in clinical software nationwide, meant Black patients appeared healthier than they actually were, delaying diagnoses of kidney disease and limiting access to transplant lists. Only in recent years, following advocacy and research published in the New England Journal of Medicine in 2023, have major health systems begun removing race from these algorithms. But the damage from years of biased calculations persists.

Pain assessment algorithms present another concerning pattern. Studies have shown that AI-driven pain scoring tools, trained on data from patient populations that were predominantly white, systematically underestimate pain in Black and Latino patients. The algorithm picks up on historical patterns where minority patients' pain complaints were taken less seriously, and it perpetuates that inequity. Patients whose pain is algorithmically scored as less severe receive less aggressive treatment, wait longer for pain relief, and suffer unnecessarily.

Even basic monitoring technology can exhibit racial bias. Pulse oximeters, devices that measure blood oxygen levels, have been shown to be significantly less accurate for patients with darker skin tones. A 2024 Science article examined how this measurement error, amplified when readings are fed into AI systems making clinical decisions, led to delayed treatment for hypoxemia in Black patients during the COVID-19 pandemic. The algorithm assumed the pulse oximeter readings were equally accurate for all patients. They weren't.

A particularly troubling aspect of algorithmic bias is its invisibility. When a human displays bias, it can be identified, challenged, and corrected. When an algorithm displays bias, it's hidden in code, obscured by claims of objectivity, and scaled across thousands of patient encounters. The system appears neutral, scientific, fair. But it's perpetuating the same inequities it inherited from biased training data.

As a patient, you can't always know if the algorithm shaping your care is biased. But you can ask questions. You can advocate for yourself. And you can demand that your individual circumstances, not population-level assumptions, drive your care.

Julie and the Algorithm That Couldn't See Pain

Here is another vignette that reveals how algorithmic rigidity can harm patients with complex conditions.

Julie had been fighting for better pain management for months. The car accident five years earlier had left her with a nerve condition that makes sustained activity excruciating. Some days are better than others, but most days she's managing baseline pain that impacts everything: how much she can work, how long she can stand, what she can do with her kids.

Her pain management had been relatively stable on a combination of physical therapy, a non-opioid pain medication, and occasional anti-inflammatory drugs. It wasn't perfect, but it worked. Then her insurance company decided to implement a new step therapy protocol for chronic pain management.

Step therapy, enforced by an algorithm, meant Julie had to try Drug A first. If that didn't work after 90 days, then Drug B. Only if both failed could she try the medication Dr. Leo Park, her pain specialist, actually wanted to prescribe for her specific condition.

The problem? Drug A had been on the market for five years. Julie had been on it five years ago when it first came out, under a different insurance plan. It had never worked for her. But the algorithm didn't know that. The records didn't talk to each other. The system saw a new insurance enrollment and assumed Drug A was a reasonable first-line option based on population data. It didn't account for Julie's previous trial and failure.

So Julie waited. Ninety days of worsening pain while she took a medication she knew wouldn't work. Meanwhile, Dr. Leo Park documented that she'd already failed this medication, submitted appeals, and requested an exception. The insurance algorithm denied the appeals automatically.

After 90 days, they moved to Drug B. Another trial period. Another 90 days of pain and frustration. Meanwhile, Julie had to call in to work more often. She had to ask her mom for help with the kids more frequently. Her quality of life deteriorated because an algorithm didn't know her history.

It took Dr. Park, the clinic staff, and persistence from Julie herself to finally escalate past the automated system to a human reviewer who actually looked at her complete medical history. Only then did they realize the algorithm was forcing her through steps she'd already taken.

Julie eventually got access to the medication Dr. Park recommended. But she'd lost six months to algorithmic inflexibility. Six months when she could have been managing her pain better, working more, being more present for her family.

The Insurance Black Box

Insurance algorithms aren't limited to step therapy. They're making life-or-death decisions every day, and most patients never know.

Insurance company AI denial patterns often rely on outdated clinical guidelines and fail to account for individual patient factors. Even more troubling: some insurance companies set target denial rates, configuring algorithmic systems to reject a certain percentage of claims regardless of medical necessity. This creates a structural barrier between patients and the care they need.

This is AI in service of extraction, not care. And patients are the ones who pay the price.

Where AI Could Have Saved Me

Here's the frustrating irony: while AI was being used to deny me care, it could have been used to prevent the worst medical error I ever experienced.

Remember the medication error I mentioned in Chapter 1? My neurologist prescribed a medication at twenty times the recommended starting dosage. Twenty times.

The pharmacy filled it without question. No one caught the error.

I took what I was prescribed, trusting that the professionals had gotten it right.

The overdose nearly killed me. I spent months hospitalized and in rehabilitation, relearning basic functions that the toxic dose had stolen from me.

And here's what haunts me: AI could have prevented this.

Modern AI-powered clinical decision support systems can perform automated safety screening on prescriptions. They check dosages against established ranges for specific medications, patient weight, age, kidney and liver function. They flag orders that fall outside safe parameters. They alert both prescribers and pharmacists when something looks wrong.

Computerized physician order entry systems with integrated AI safety checks can reduce medication errors significantly. AI-enabled dosage range checking catches prescribing errors in a small but important percentage of all orders—errors that would otherwise reach patients and potentially cause harm.

My prescription was twenty times too high. Any reasonably designed AI safety system should have caught that instantly. It should have stopped the order before it was ever sent to the pharmacy. It should have alerted my neurologist that something was catastrophically wrong.

But it didn't. Because either the system didn't have AI safety screening, or it had it but someone overrode the alert without investigating, or the AI wasn't configured correctly to catch dosing errors of this magnitude.

In the end, no one admitted anything was wrong. I was left to bear the consequences of a preventable error that cost me months of my life.

So here's the paradox I live with: AI denied me a medication I needed because an algorithm said I hadn't followed the right steps. But AI could have saved me from a medication error that nearly killed me, if anyone had bothered to implement the safety systems that already exist.

The technology to help patients is here. We're just not using it consistently or wisely.

The Predictability Problem

Remember what I said in Chapter 1? The healthcare system loves predictability. It's designed for patterns, not exceptions.

AI amplifies this tendency. Algorithms learn from past patterns to predict future outcomes. They're incredibly good at recognizing what they've seen before. They're terrible at handling what they haven't.

This creates a particular problem for patients with chronic, complex conditions. People like me.

Take those step therapy algorithms I mentioned: the ones that say you must try Drug A, then Drug B, then Drug C before you can access the treatment your doctor actually prescribed. In theory, they make sense. Why not try less expensive options first? Why not follow established treatment guidelines?

But theory assumes your condition is predictable. It assumes you fit the pattern the algorithm was trained on. It assumes the standard pathway will work for you.

When you have a complex chronic condition, none of those assumptions hold. You might have drug sensitivities that make Drug A dangerous for you. You might have failed Drug B three years ago with a different doctor in a different system, but the algorithm doesn't know that because the records don't talk to each other. You might have complicating factors, other medications, other conditions, genetic variations, that mean the standard pathway won't work.

But the algorithm doesn't care about complexity. It cares about matching patterns. And if you don't match the pattern, you're out of luck.

This is when you need to speak up. This is when you need to request human oversight and review.

The Sepsis Algorithm That Cried Wolf

The predictability problem becomes dangerous when algorithms are implemented without understanding their limitations. Consider what happened at a major hospital system that deployed an AI tool designed to predict sepsis, a life-threatening condition that requires immediate treatment.

The algorithm analyzed patient vital signs, lab values, and other data in real-time, alerting nurses when it detected patterns suggesting early sepsis. In theory, this should save lives by catching the condition before it becomes critical.

In practice, the system started alerting on approximately 40% of all patients admitted to the hospital. The vast majority, over 95%, were false positives. Patients who had slightly abnormal vital signs for benign reasons. Patients whose lab values triggered the algorithm's thresholds but who showed no clinical signs of infection. Patients the algorithm flagged as high-risk who were actually stable.

What happened next is predictable if you understand human behavior: alert fatigue. When nurses are told that nearly half of their patients are at risk for a life-threatening condition, but almost all of those alerts turn out to be false alarms, they stop trusting the system. The alerts become noise. They learn to dismiss them.

And then one patient who actually was developing sepsis got lost in the noise. The algorithm alerted. The nurse, overwhelmed by constant false alarms, didn't prioritize the warning. By the time the patient's deterioration became obvious without the AI, valuable hours had been lost.

Multiple hospitals have experienced serious problems with sepsis prediction algorithms. Poorly calibrated AI systems, implemented with insufficient testing and validation, created more risk than benefit. The technology worked in the controlled research environment. It failed in the messy reality of clinical care.

The problem wasn't that AI can't help predict sepsis. It was that this particular implementation didn't account for the complexity and variability of real patients. It didn't consider the human factors: how clinicians would respond to constant alerts. It prioritized sensitivity, catching every possible case, over specificity, accurately distinguishing true risk from false alarms.

This is what happens when AI is implemented without adequate oversight, testing, and adjustment for real-world conditions. The algorithm became worse than useless. It became dangerous.

Stop, Drop, and Reconsider

When an algorithm is making decisions about your care and something doesn't feel right, when the recommendation doesn't match your reality, when you're being forced down a pathway that doesn't make sense for your situation, when you're told "the computer says" and it contradicts what you know about your own body, it's time to make the system pause.

Stop: Halt the automated process. Don't just accept the algorithmic decision.

Drop: Set aside the assumption that the computer must be right. Algorithms are tools, not oracles.

Reconsider: Demand human review. Ask for an exception. Insist that someone with medical training and the ability to understand context look at your specific situation.

This isn't being difficult. This isn't rejecting technology. This is recognizing that AI systems are designed for the typical case, and you might not be typical. You might be the exception that proves why we still need human judgment.

The system loves predictability because predictability is efficient. But your health isn't about efficiency. It's about effectiveness. And sometimes effective care requires the system to stop, drop its automated assumptions, and reconsider.

What You Need to Know

AI in healthcare isn't inherently good or bad. It's a tool. Like any tool, it can help or harm depending on how it's designed, implemented, and governed.

The AI that translated my MRI report? Helpful. It gave me understanding and reduced my anxiety while I waited for my appointment. That's AI serving the patient.

The AI that could have caught my medication error? Life-saving. That's AI as a safety net, catching human mistakes before they reach patients.

The AI that denied me necessary medication? Harmful. That's AI prioritizing cost containment over clinical judgment, with no human oversight to recognize when the algorithm doesn't fit the patient.

The difference between these scenarios isn't the technology itself. It's who's in control, what the goals are, and whether there's human judgment in the loop.

And here's what you need to understand as a patient: most of the time, you won't know AI is involved unless you ask.

When AI Actually Helped: Mary's Discovery

Because this chapter has focused heavily on AI failures and harms, I want to share a story where AI genuinely helped a patient, when it was used transparently, appropriately, and in the service of better care.

Mary's mother's Alzheimer's had been progressing, and the worry was eating into everything: sleep, concentration, patience. Mary's mom still lives at home, but the disease is progressing, and Mary manages most of her medical appointments, medication schedules, and health decisions.

Last year, at her mother's annual physical, Dr. Susan Chang suggested implementing an AI-assisted fall-risk assessment. The system uses data from wearable devices, activity tracking, and clinical history to predict which older adults are at high risk for falls. Falls are serious for aging adults, particularly those with cognitive decline, and early identification can trigger preventive interventions.

Mary was skeptical. But Dr. Chang explained the system clearly: it would analyze her mom's data, flag concerning patterns, and Dr. Chang would review the results to recommend modifications to her home, changes in her mother's routine, and follow-up monitoring.

The algorithm flagged that Mary's mom's nighttime activity patterns had changed. She was getting up more frequently at night, unsteadily, without the usual pre-awakening time. This pattern suggested increasing falls risk at night. When Dr. Chang reviewed the data, she discussed it with Mary, and they made several changes: nightlights in the hallway, a bedside commode to reduce nighttime bathroom trips, adjustments to her mother's evening medications to improve nighttime stability.

Three months later, her mother hadn't had a fall. Previously, she'd been falling roughly once every couple of months.

What made this different from the problematic AI stories? Several things: Mary's mom knew AI was being used, Dr. Chang explained the process upfront, and consent was part of the conversation. A human physician reviewed the AI findings and made the final clinical judgment. The AI was used as a decision support tool, not a decision-making replacement. The system was designed to help patients, not reduce costs or limit care.

This is what good AI implementation looks like. AI-assisted fall-risk prediction in older adults is now more accurate than human-only assessment, catching early changes that prevent serious injuries. But the key is how it's implemented: transparent, collaborative, with human oversight.

AI doesn't have to be invisible and harmful. It can be visible and helpful. The difference is whether the system is designed with patients' interests at the center.

The Consent Problem

Mary's story raises an important question: should patients have to consent to AI being used in their care?

Right now, the answer is almost always no. You don't consent to the triage algorithm that determines how quickly you're seen in the

ER. You don't consent to the insurance algorithm that decides whether your treatment is covered. You don't consent to the risk prediction algorithm that influences your hospital care. These systems are implemented at the institutional level, and individual patient consent isn't part of the equation.

Think about this. When a doctor recommends surgery, you have the right to understand the risks and benefits. You can say yes or no. But when an algorithm makes a coverage decision or recommends a treatment pathway? You usually have no idea it's happening. No chance to consent. No chance to opt out.

Some experts argue patients should be informed when AI is being used and should have the right to request human-only decisions. Others say that's impractical, since AI is so embedded in healthcare now that you can't easily extract it.

But even if you can't opt out entirely, shouldn't you at least know when AI is influencing your care? Shouldn't you be able to ask what data it's using? Whether it's been tested for bias? How often it's wrong?

Some healthcare systems are starting to disclose when AI tools are involved in your care. But these are voluntary, not required. Most patients still encounter AI without any disclosure or chance to question it.

It comes down to this: you have the right to make informed decisions about your own care. But how can you make informed decisions when you don't know an algorithm is involved? How can you have any say over a process you can't see?

I don't have all the answers. But I know this: when AI operates invisibly, without your knowledge or consent, it undermines everything patient-centered care is supposed to be about. You need transparency. You need the right to know. And you need the ability to challenge algorithmic decisions when they don't make sense for your situation.

The Questions to Ask

So how do you make the invisible visible? How do you uncover the algorithms already making decisions about your care?

You ask.

When you're told you don't qualify for something, ask: "Is this decision being made by a person or a computer system?"

When your insurance denies coverage, ask: "What algorithm or criteria determined this? Can a human review my specific circumstances?"

When you're given a risk score or triage decision, ask: "How was this calculated? What factors did the system consider? What factors might it have missed about my specific situation?"

When a treatment pathway is recommended, ask: "Is this based on an algorithm or clinical guidelines? How much flexibility is there to adjust for my individual circumstances?"

You won't always get clear answers. Sometimes the person you're asking doesn't know themselves. The algorithm is buried in systems they don't control or fully understand. But asking the question accomplishes something important: it makes visible what was invisible.

It signals that you're paying attention. That you expect transparency. That you're not just a passive recipient of whatever the computer spits out.

And sometimes, not always, but sometimes, asking these questions opens doors. It prompts someone to request an exception. To escalate to a human reviewer. To consider whether the algorithm actually fits your case.

The Danger of DIY AI

I need to circle back to that MRI report translation, because there's something important we need to talk about.

More and more patients are using AI tools to interpret their medical reports, research their symptoms, and try to make sense of complex health information. I did it. You might do it. It's becoming common.

But we need to be honest about the risks.

When I fed my MRI report into an AI tool, that tool had no context about my medical history, my symptoms, my previous imaging, or what my doctor was looking for. It gave me a general interpretation of medical terminology. It helped me understand the words. But it couldn't tell me what those findings meant for my specific situation.

AI can explain medical jargon. It cannot replace medical judgment.

It can help you formulate better questions for your doctor. It cannot diagnose you.

It can reduce your anxiety by making complex reports more understandable. But it can also increase anxiety if it highlights something concerning without the context to know whether it's actually worrisome in your case.

So if you use AI tools to understand your health information, and I think there's value in doing so, do it with eyes open:

Share the AI interpretation with your doctor. Let them confirm, clarify, or correct what the AI told you.

Don't make medical decisions based solely on AI output. Use it to inform your questions, not replace professional guidance.

Be cautious about what information you feed into AI tools. Some have privacy implications. Your medical information is sensitive.

Remember that AI tools vary in quality and accuracy. Not all are created equal. Some are trained on better data than others.

AI as a tool for understanding? Valuable. AI as a replacement for your doctor? Dangerous.

The Path Forward

What I want you to take away from this chapter:

AI is already deeply embedded in your healthcare. You encounter it far more often than you realize. Most of the time, it's invisible.

Sometimes that AI helps you. It catches errors, coordinates care, flags potential problems, translates complex information.

Sometimes it harms you. It denies necessary care, forces you down inappropriate pathways, misses patterns that don't match its training data.

The difference between helpful and harmful AI isn't the technology itself. It's how it's designed, who controls it, what its goals are, and whether there's meaningful human oversight.

As a patient, your power lies in making the invisible visible. In asking whether computers or humans are making decisions. In demanding explanations. In requesting exceptions when the algorithm doesn't fit your situation.

And in knowing when to say: Stop. Drop your automated assumptions. Reconsider my specific circumstances.

Because the system loves predictability. But you're not a predictable pattern to be matched. You're a complex human being with a unique story.

And sometimes the most important thing you can do is remind the system of that.

In the next chapter, we'll explore the positive side of this equation: how AI, when used correctly, can actually amplify your voice and help you reclaim partnership in your care. But first, you need to see the AI that's already there. You need to make it visible.

Because you can't govern what you can't see.

Questions Worth Sitting With

Before moving to the next chapter, reflect on these questions:

Have you ever been told "the computer says" or "the system shows" about your healthcare? What was that experience like?

Can you think of a time when an algorithm might have been making decisions about your care without you knowing?

Have you ever used AI tools (ChatGPT, Google's medical search, etc.) to research your symptoms or understand medical reports? What did you learn? Did you share it with your doctor?

Have you experienced a situation where you didn't fit the standard treatment pathway? How did that get resolved?

At your next appointment or insurance interaction, what question will you ask to make AI decision-making more visible?

Write down your thoughts. In the next chapter, we'll explore how to harness AI as a tool for patient empowerment rather than just experiencing it as an invisible force.

QUICK TOOL: AI Decision-Making Questions Card

Keep this card in your wallet, on your phone, or save it on your device. Use it at your next healthcare visit or insurance interaction.

1. Is this decision being made by an AI algorithm, or a person?
2. What criteria or guidelines is this decision based on?
3. Has my specific medical history been reviewed, or is this a blanket policy decision?
4. Can someone look at my individual circumstances and make an exception?
5. What happens if I disagree with this decision? What's my appeal process?
6. If this is an algorithmic decision, can I speak to a human reviewer?
7. What are the next steps if I want to challenge this decision?

Remember: You have the right to understand how decisions about your care are being made. Don't be afraid to ask.

4

———

MY BRAIN IS BUFFERING

Finding Your Second Brain - You've been following Sarah's journey; she's 32, living with Type 2 diabetes, and she sits in her endocrinologist's office trying to write down what Dr. Cara Webster just explained about her blood sugar patterns. Her hand is moving, but her brain has checked out. She's exhausted from work. She's overwhelmed by the flood of information. She's scared that she's already messing this up.

As she leaves the office, Sarah looks at the notes she tried to take. The handwriting is shaky. Half of it doesn't make sense. Did Dr. Webster say to check her blood sugar before meals or after? Was it supposed to be twice a day or four times? And that thing about carbs ... was she supposed to count them or avoid them?

She's not confused because she doesn't care. She's confused because being sick steals your bandwidth. Because there's too much to hold at once. Because nobody, not her doctor, not the system, not even her own brain, is giving her the one thing she actually needs right now: a partner to help her remember what matters and ask the right questions at the next visit.

Nobody likes being sick. Nobody likes feeling like something is wrong in their own body. If you've read this far, you know that feeling. Overwhelmed. Confused. Afraid. The distracted doctor. The invisible algorithms that may be shaping decisions. The insurance company that says no before a human ever really looks.

It all comes from uncertainty. And if I'm being honest, it can turn into something worse: the fear that nobody truly understands.

Maybe you're reading this because you have a health issue. Managing diabetes. Living with chronic pain. In the midst of cancer treatment. Or dealing with heart disease, or maybe a combination of conditions. Maybe you're reading because you're scared of getting sick: family history, new test results, the clock suddenly louder than it used to be. Or maybe you just want more control. Sleep better. Eat smarter. Understand your body more clearly.

Whatever brought you here, here's what I've learned: the tools that help me survive a neurological condition that can be debilitating are the same kinds of tools that can help many people take control of their own health circumstances. Whether you're in crisis or trying to prevent one. Whether you're managing multiple medications or trying to understand a new test or treatment that the doctor has ordered. You have options.

However, then came the moment that changed everything for me. Not a dramatic moment. Not a breakthrough or a miracle. Just a quiet, devastating realization as I sat in my specialist's office, years into this journey. So sure, I had options, but I also had to accept that life was changing.

Things may improve. But I'll never be cured.

I have a chronic medical condition.

When I say chronic, I mean it's not going away. Ever. Despite how frustrated I get.

Let me explain the difference. If I fall and break my ankle, that's acute. They put me in a cast to hold the bones in place. Six to eight weeks later, they take the cast off and I'm healed. Problem solved.

Chronic is different. Chronic means there's no timeline for healing. No cast that comes off. No "you're all better now." It's permanent.

My condition? A bleed in my brain from a fall. The damage from that injury, combined with a medication error, turned it into something I'll live with for the rest of my life. Not a problem to solve. Not a prescription that suddenly fixes everything. A companion. For life.

When that reality settled in, I realized something else: I needed help. Long-term help. Not just doctor visits every six to eight weeks. Not just medication reminders. I needed something, or someone, to walk with me through this. To help me keep context. To help me find resources. To help me ask better questions.

I needed a second brain. Because mine wasn't always going to be there for me.

What I Mean by "Second Brain"

I want to explain what I mean by "second brain," because I'm not talking about something technical or complicated. I'm talking about a partner that helps you think. One that remembers what you might forget. One that helps connect dots that are hard to see when you're overwhelmed, exhausted, or scared.

It's like having a really smart friend who's always available. Who never gets impatient. Who can hold onto the details of your health journey even when you can't?

Whether you're dealing with the cognitive effects of a brain injury like me, or chemo brain, or medication side effects, or chronic fatigue, or the plain stress of being sick, or even if you're healthy but drowning in conflicting nutrition advice and fitness trends, we all have moments when thinking clearly feels out of reach. Moments when there's too much information and not enough understanding. Moments when we need help stepping back and seeing the bigger picture.

That's when having a thinking partner matters most.

The Science Behind AI as Your Partner

When I started using AI (artificial intelligence) to help manage my health, I had a nagging worry: was I just telling myself a nice story? Was this actually helping, or was it basically a placebo wrapped in convenience? And if it *was* helping, was there any research that matched what I was experiencing?

What I found is more nuanced, and more human, than I expected. The best evidence doesn't say, "AI improves your health in a simple, guaranteed way." What it *does* support is something quieter, but still meaningful: certain patient-facing tools can help people feel more oriented, more prepared, and less alone in the long, exhausting stretch between appointments. In other words, AI can function like scaffolding. Supporting your memory. Your attention. Your ability to communicate. Especially when illness steals your bandwidth.

Start with what clinicians often fear. A multicenter randomized controlled trial of a symptom-checker app used by self-referred walk-in patients in the emergency department specifically examined whether the tool would make patients more anxious or less trusting of clinicians. It didn't. Anxiety and trust did not worsen, even though the tool didn't magically improve satisfaction with the visit. Many patients and clinicians still reported that it felt helpful. (Schmieding et al., 2025, JMIR).

That "didn't worsen" finding matters because it answers a real clinical question: will patient-facing AI inflame panic or damage the relationship? In that study, it didn't.

OTHER RESEARCH ASKED A DIFFERENT QUESTION. Not "Did the AI get the diagnosis right?" but "Did talking to the AI actually help the person?"

They looked at things like: Did you understand what might be wrong with you? Did you feel more confident about what to do next? Did it make you less anxious, or more anxious? Did you feel more in control of your health situation?

These are the things you can actually feel. The things that matter to you when you're scared at 2 AM wondering if you should go to the emergency room or wait until morning.

The point wasn't that the AI had to be perfect. The point was whether the conversation helped you understand what you were dealing with and figure out your next step with less panic and more clarity.

Looking across many studies, symptom checkers work best when users trust them, find them easy to use, feel safe using them, and use them in the right context. The clinical evidence base is growing rapidly.

But here's where I think the deeper point lives, and where "partner" becomes more than a metaphor.

Health issues can make you feel very lonely. Not just emotionally, but cognitively. You can be surrounded by people and still feel like you're carrying a private, exhausting mental load: remembering symptoms, tracking medications, keeping timelines straight, trying to translate medical language into something you can live inside. Loneliness isn't just a mood. It's associated with chronic illness and health outcomes in measurable ways.

Research shows that loneliness and chronic health problems are deeply connected. When you're lonely, your health gets worse. When you're sick, you often become more isolated and lonely. They feed into each other, creating a cycle that's hard to break.

This is also where older, very well-established research on patient empowerment and follow-through becomes relevant. A large systematic review in PLOS ONE found that empowerment-related factors like self-efficacy and an internal sense of control are consistently associated with better medication adherence across studies. In plain language: when patients feel more capable and supported, they're more likely to do the hard, boring, repetitive things health requires. (Náfrádi et al., 2017).

That doesn't mean "information makes you a perfect patient." It means something simpler: support changes what you're able to carry.

Now comes the philosophical layer, and the part that feels closest to my actual life.

In most modern healthcare, your clinicians are not available at midnight. They're not sitting with you on the anxious Tuesday when the fog rolls in and you can't hold onto a thought long enough to finish a sentence. They're not there when you need to turn a week of scattered symptoms into a coherent story. They shouldn't be. They have other patients, other constraints, and the limits of the system are real.

AI can't replace human care. It can't love you. It can't examine you. It can't make decisions for you. But it can sometimes do something that is surprisingly rare in healthcare: it can stay with you. Consistently. Patiently. Without time pressure. Long enough to help you think.

That "staying with you" is not just poetic language. Conversational AI systems designed for companionship can reduce loneliness in some settings and populations, depending on whether users feel heard and understood.

At the same time, there's a caution here: heavy emotional reliance on AI may correlate with greater loneliness or emotional dependence for some users, depending on how and how much the tool is used.

Both things can be true: AI can relieve loneliness for some people in some moments, and still carry risks if it becomes a substitute for human connection.

That's why the healthiest frame, especially for patients, is "partner," not "provider."

That's also where my lived experience lines up with what the research *actually* supports. The AI didn't "diagnose" me. It helped me organize my reality well enough to bring it to the right human being. It didn't announce a drug interaction like a courtroom verdict. It helped me gather my medication list, clarify what I was noticing, and ask my neurologist a sharper question. It didn't replace clinical judgment. It supported the work of clinical judgment by making the input, my story, more coherent.

And here's the difference that matters most to me: context and continuity.

When you Google symptoms at 2 a.m., you get an anxious slot machine: possibilities ranging from "you're fine" to "catastrophe," with no memory of who you are. Your history. Your medications. What you've already been evaluated for. Or what your clinician told you last time. A well-bounded AI assistant, used over time, can be useful in a different way: not to tell you what's "wrong," but to help you hold onto context. Your baseline. Your timeline. Your patterns. Your questions. Your own words. It can help you organize what you're noticing into something clearer to track and share, so you can ask, "Is this change something we should talk about?" or "Could this be related to my medication?" Instead of trying to decide the answer at midnight, you're preparing the right information for the right human conversation. And showing up with a coherent story, less scattered, more specific, can make the visit more productive.

To be clear, none of this replaces medical expertise. But it can fill a critical gap: the space between appointments. The questions that appear at midnight. The details you forget the moment you're sitting under fluorescent lights in an exam room. That's where "AI as a second brain" can make a real difference. Quietly. Steadily. Safely.

Sarah's Follow-Up

A week after her appointment, Sarah sits at home with the appointment summary her clinic sent her. It's detailed, but it's still full of medical terminology. She pulls up her phone and opens a voice-activated AI assistant. "I got this letter from my doctor about my diabetes, but I don't understand it. Can you read it and explain what it means in plain language?"

The AI reads it. Summarizes it. Explains what each recommendation actually means for her day-to-day life. And then Sarah asks the question that matters most: "What should I ask Dr. Webster about at my next visit to make sure I'm doing this right?"

The AI helps her generate three concrete questions, written in her own words. When she goes back to Dr. Webster with that list, the conversation is different. Sarah isn't confused and overwhelmed. She's prepared. And Dr. Webster, seeing that Sarah has engaged with her own care, spends more time answering those questions carefully.

This is what AI as a second brain looks like when it's working: not replacing the clinician. Supporting the partnership between patient and clinician.

The Medication That Shouldn't Have Been

Let me tell you about the moment I realized AI could be more than just a research tool. It could actually help me be a better patient.

My primary care physician prescribed a new medication. Routine appointment, routine prescription. He wrote it out, told me to start it, sent me on my way. A few weeks later, I mentioned it to my neurologist, the world-leading specialist who manages my seizures and neurological complications.

He paused. Just for a second. Then gave me a word of caution. Not stern. Not detailed. Just a caution. He didn't elaborate. He didn't tell me to stop taking it. He just said to be careful.

Now, I don't know about you, but when a specialist who specializes in exactly what's wrong with me gives me "a word of caution" about a medication, I need to understand what that means. What was he cautioning me about? Why didn't he elaborate? Should I be worried? Should I stop taking it?

So I did what I'd been learning to do. I turned to AI.

I described my specific situation. The TBI. The seizures. The other medications I was taking. I asked about this new prescription. What could the concerns be? What interactions might exist? What side effects should I watch for?

The answer made my stomach drop. This medication could have serious short-term consequences that would only get worse over time. What really scared me was that the side effects could last even if you stopped taking the medication. The interactions with my other medications could amplify the risks. Getting off it could be extremely difficult. This wasn't a minor concern. This was a very big problem.

Armed with this information, I went back to my neurologist. Not to tell him what AI said. Not to contradict his expertise. But to ask the right question: "Is this a medication I should avoid? Are you recommending that I don't take this?"

His demeanor changed completely. "Yes," he said firmly. "I've seen people on this medication. It's terrible to get off of. There are terrible consequences. You should not take this medication."

I need you to catch what just happened there. My neurologist used the word "consequences." I hadn't heard him use that word very often. This wasn't academic. This was serious.

The AI didn't replace my neurologist's judgment. It didn't give me medical advice I followed blindly. What it did was help me understand a vague caution enough to ask the right follow-up question. It bridged the gap between "be careful" and "you should not take this medication."

Later, I told my primary care physician who prescribed the medication, "I've decided not to take that medication." That's it. No explanation. No mention of AI or my neurologist. Just: I've decided not to take it. I was sovereign.

This past summer, that same primary care physician threatened to fire me as a patient because I was questioning his care. This wasn't the first time I'd questioned his prescriptions. It was a pattern. And apparently, he'd had enough of me asking questions.

But here's what I learned: AI didn't make me a difficult patient. It made me a better one. It gave me the tools to advocate for myself without being reckless. It helped me ask questions that protected me.

Pain That Won't Sit Still

Some mornings Julie can barely get out of bed. The chronic radiating pain doesn't care that she has two teenagers to feed and a job to hold down. One day it's her lower back. Another day, it's her shoulders and neck. Some mornings she wakes up fine. Other mornings she's in tears before her feet hit the floor.

Her pain management specialist, Dr. Leo Park, keeps asking her the same questions at each visit: What's been bothering you? When does the pain get worse? What makes it better? Julie tries to answer, but she can't remember the specific days. She can't recall what she was doing when it flared. Was it worse last month or two months ago?

So Julie started using an AI-powered pain tracker. Every evening, she spends two minutes logging: Where does it hurt? What's the pain level from 1 to 10? What did she do today that might have made it worse or better? What did she eat? How did she sleep?

Three months later, when Julie went back to Dr. Park, she brought her summary. The tracker had found a pattern Julie hadn't noticed herself: her pain flared predictably two days after she skipped her physical therapy routine. It also got worse when she stayed up past 11 p.m.

Dr. Park adjusted her treatment plan based on this real data from Julie's actual life. He prescribed better sleep coaching. He validated the importance of her physical therapy. He added a small medication adjustment to help with the flares that happened despite her best efforts.

This is what AI as a second brain means for someone with chronic pain. It's not replacing Dr. Park's expertise. It's giving him the information he needs to help Julie make changes that actually work for her life.

Collaboration, Not Contradiction

Another time, I had an MRI of my brain. When the report came back, it was full of medical terminology I didn't understand. Phrases like "encephalomalacia" and "gliosis" and measurements of ventricles. I could look up each term individually, but I wouldn't understand what it meant as a whole. What was the bigger picture? What should I be asking about?

I used Gemini to help me translate the report into plain language.

Not to diagnose myself. Not to second-guess my doctors. But to prepare for the conversation with my specialist. To understand what questions I should ask.

When I met with my neurologist, I shared what I'd learned. Not as a challenge. Not as "look what I found on the internet." But as a starting point for discussion. "I used AI to help me understand my MRI report. Here's what I think it's saying. Can you help me understand it more?"

And together, we walked through it. He explained it in more detail. He put it in context of my overall condition. He answered questions I wouldn't have known to ask without that AI translation.

This is what I mean by collaboration. I wasn't undermining his expertise. I was preparing myself to receive it. The AI empowered me to be a better participant in my own care.

Think about it this way: if you went to the library and researched your medical condition before seeing your doctor, that book wouldn't become your provider. It would just be a point of reference to help you understand the situation better. AI works the same way, except it can answer your follow-up questions, understand your specific context, and help you see patterns you might miss.

Mary's Double Burden

Mary was disappearing into her mother's care. Not dramatically—no one noticed—but slowly, the way a candle burns down while you're reading in another room. Every week, Mary is managing her mother's doctor appointments, medication schedule, specialist referrals, and memory loss. She's also trying to keep her own health stable. Her own cardiologist appointments. Her own blood pressure medication. Her own annual physicals.

One day, Mary realized she hadn't been to her own doctor in two years. She'd been so focused on her mother's care that she'd let her own health slide into the background.

She started using an AI-powered personal health organizer. It sends her reminders when she has appointments coming up. It helps her keep track of her mother's medications and appointments in one place. When her primary care physician, Dr. Susan Chang, asks how Mary is managing stress, Mary can show her the tracker. It's real data about Mary's own sleep, exercise, and stress levels.

Dr. Chang doesn't dismiss Mary's self-reported stress. She sees it reflected in Mary's blood pressure numbers and sleep logs. Together, they make a plan. Mary gets a referral to a therapist who specializes in caregiver burnout. She also gets a conversation with her mother's care team about whether they can coordinate more, so Mary isn't calling three different offices every week.

This is what AI as a second brain means for someone juggling their own health and someone else's care. It's not a replacement for human attention. It's a way to make sure that you, the caregiver, don't get lost in the process.

More Than Search: Understanding

Here's the thing about AI that makes it different from just Googling your symptoms at 2 a.m. I've done it, no judgment. It's not about finding information. It's about understanding it comprehensively.

When I was navigating my TBI and seizures and four different neurologists, I trained my AI, specifically ChatGPT, to understand my condition in a special, dedicated project. What I'd been through. How does it make me feel? What medications am I on? My history. My concerns. There is a word of caution about this. I am sharing personal information that I am willing to share. You will want to consider this when using any tool that does not provide clear, private, HIPAA-compliant sharing and storage of information.

So when I ask a follow-up question weeks later, it has context. It knows about my multiple conditions. It knows I have complex neurological events. It knows I've seen multiple neurologists and other specialists. It's not starting from zero every time. It's building on what we've discussed before.

Last week, it referenced something I told it last month. That kind of continuity matters when you're managing a chronic condition and your own memory isn't always reliable.

But here's what I learned the hard way: this is a partnership that requires your communication. The AI can't read your mind. It can't know what you're actually doing unless you tell it. If I research a treatment option and decide not to pursue it, I need to tell the AI that. Otherwise, next time we talk, it might assume I went that direction.

I've actually had Claude tell me, "Dan, you're pushing too hard. You've been asking me too many questions. You need to take a break." No other AI tool has done that. The others will just keep going and going and going, and frankly, they become less and less effective the longer you talk with them. But Claude recognized when I was overdoing it and told me to step away from the computer.

That's the kind of assistant I needed. Not just a search engine. A partner that could help me see when I was spiraling.

Privacy Note: Anonymize Before You Share

Before pasting any health information into AI tools like ChatGPT or Claude, remove all identifying details. Replace your name with "Patient X," your age with a range ("mid-40s"), and avoid specific dates or locations. These tools are powerful, but they're not HIPAA-compliant. Treat them like you're talking to a smart friend at a coffee shop—helpful, but not your doctor, and not entitled to your full medical record.

Practical AI Tools You Can Use Today

When I talk about using AI as a second brain, people often ask: "What exactly should I use? Where do I start?" That's a fair question. The AI landscape changes rapidly, but let me walk you through some practical categories and tools that exist right now. I don't endorse any of these, so I'm sharing them simply for your consideration.

Conversational AI Assistants

These are the tools I use most: Claude, ChatGPT, and Google's Gemini. Each has strengths. Claude tends to be more conversational and cautious, often flagging when it thinks you should talk to a doctor. ChatGPT has a massive knowledge base and can summarize research quickly. Gemini integrates well with Google services and can help you organize health information across different platforms.

The key with any of these: have extended conversations. Don't just ask one question and leave. Build a relationship over time. Tell the AI about your condition, your medications, your concerns. Then keep that conversation going. These tools remember context within a conversation thread. Use that to your advantage.

Symptom and Health Trackers

Apps like Bearable, Flaredown, and Manage My Pain use AI to help you track symptoms and identify patterns. You log how you're feeling, what you ate, how you slept, what medications you took. Over time, the AI looks for correlations. "Your headaches seem to occur most often two days after you reduce your sleep below six hours." That kind of insight is invisible when you're just living day to day.

These aren't diagnostic tools. They're pattern-recognition tools. They help you see your health more clearly so you can have better conversations with your doctor.

Medical Document Translation

This is where conversational AI really shines. When you get lab results, imaging reports, or medical records, you can upload them or paste them into Claude or ChatGPT and ask for a plain-language explanation. "What is this report telling me? What should I ask my doctor about?"

I do this routinely. Every MRI report, every blood test, every specialist note. I don't accept the AI's interpretation as fact. I use it to prepare questions for my doctor. It transforms me from a passive recipient of information to an active participant in understanding what's happening in my body.

Research Summarization

When I find a research study about my neurological condition, I often paste it into Gemini and ask for a summary focused on what's relevant to my specific situation. "What does this study mean for someone with post-traumatic epilepsy? Are there any findings that would change how I should think about my treatment?"

This saves me hours. I can scan multiple studies in the time it would take me to carefully read one. Then, if something seems important, I can dive deeper into that specific area.

A Word of Caution About Health Apps

Not all health AI is created equal. Some apps make diagnostic claims they can't back up. Some sell your health data. Some provide advice that's overly general or even dangerous.

Stick with established tools. Read the privacy policies. Understand that these are assistive tools, not replacement tools. They help you understand, track, and communicate. They don't diagnose, treat, or cure.

And always, always, verify important information with your actual healthcare providers. AI is your research assistant and thinking partner. Your doctor is your doctor.

Your Second Brain, Your Journey

Your situation is different from mine. You might not have a neurologist. Maybe you have an endocrinologist managing your diabetes. Or an oncologist guiding your cancer treatment. Or a cardiologist monitoring your heart. Maybe you don't have a specialist at all. You're just trying to figure out why you're exhausted all the time. Or how to lose weight. Or whether that pain in your knee is something to worry about.

The specifics don't matter. What matters is this: whether you're sick or trying to stay healthy, you deserve tools that help you understand your body better. You deserve to be heard. You deserve to be a partner in your own health.

The Conductor and the Orchestra. Here's how I think about my role now: I'm the conductor of an orchestra. I have all these various instruments. My primary care physician. My neurologist. My other specialists. My test results. My research. My AI assistant. My role isn't to play all the instruments myself. It's to bring the strengths of each one together.

Because I'm the opera. I'm the performance. And I need everyone to work with me to produce the best possible outcome.

Before I see my doctor, I prepare. I use AI to help me think through what questions I should ask. "Tell me what I don't know. Tell me what questions I should be asking." Then I go to my appointment with a notebook, questions already written out. Ready to get the most out of those fifteen minutes.

I've had appointments that wrap up in five to seven minutes because I'm so focused. We go through all my questions, he answers them all, and I'm ready to leave. But here's what's interesting: sometimes my doctor will say, "Oh no, Dan, we have more time. Let's talk a little bit more." By being organized, I actually get more out of the appointment than if I'd just gone in and adapted to his flow.

Then, after the appointment, I go back to my AI partner. "Okay, I got these answers. What does this mean in context? What should I be thinking about? What follow-up questions might I need to ask next time?"

This cycle, prepare, engage, reflect, has made me a better patient. Not because I'm smarter or more informed than my doctors. But because I'm a better partner in my own care.

My Neurologist Gets It

My neurologist, the world-leading specialist who manages my seizures, is open to this. He actually likes that I do this kind of research. I'll share what I'm learning with him, and he'll tell me, "Yeah, that's on track for your situation, Dan," or "That's not going to really fit for you."

And that's what I need. I need AI to broaden my understanding. To help me learn things from a global perspective. Then I need my neurologist to pinpoint: "Okay, here's something to be concerned about," or "Here's something that doesn't apply to you, don't worry about it."

AI helps me see the forest. My doctor helps me navigate the specific trees I need to pay attention to.

I can spend thirty minutes researching a new study about TBI recovery or seizure management. AI will summarize a fifteen-to-twenty-page report, help me understand the conclusions, show me what additional studies say, explain what it all means. Then my neurologist helps me understand whether any of it actually applies to me.

This is the model I wish every patient could experience. Not doctors who feel threatened by informed patients. Not algorithms that make decisions without explanation. But genuine partnership where AI amplifies your voice and doctors welcome the conversation.

When NOT to Use AI: Boundaries and Limitations

I've spent this entire chapter telling you how AI can help you manage your health. Now I need to tell you when it can't. When it shouldn't. When you need to put down the phone and talk to a real human being.

Because here's the truth: AI is a powerful tool, but it's not a substitute for medical care. It's not a replacement for human judgment. And there are clear lines you should never cross.

Medical Emergencies

If you're having chest pain, difficulty breathing, severe bleeding, signs of a stroke, or any other acute medical emergency, do not ask an AI what to do. Call 911. Go to the emergency room. Get immediate medical care.

AI can't examine you. It can't run tests. It can't see what's actually happening in your body. In an emergency, minutes matter. Don't waste them typing questions into a chatbot.

I learned this the hard way. I've had seizures where my first instinct was to try to figure out what triggered it, to analyze it, to understand it. But when you're having a medical crisis, understanding comes later. Safety comes first.

Diagnosis and Treatment Decisions

AI should never diagnose you. It should never tell you what treatment to pursue. It can help you understand options, research possibilities, and formulate questions. But the actual decision-making must happen with a qualified healthcare provider who can examine you, order appropriate tests, and apply clinical judgment.

When that medication issue came up for me, I didn't stop taking it because AI said it was dangerous. I asked my neurologist. He made the call. AI informed my question, but it didn't make the decision.

This matters more than you might think. AI is trained on patterns from millions of cases. But you're not a pattern. You're a specific person with a specific medical history and specific circumstances. Your doctor can see those nuances. AI can't.

MENTAL HEALTH CRISES

If you're experiencing suicidal thoughts, severe depression, panic attacks, or other mental health crises, AI is not the answer. You need human help immediately.

- **Call a crisis hotline.** In the US, call or text 988. Outside the US, search online for "crisis hotline" plus your country name to find your local resource.
- **Talk to a therapist or counselor.** If you already have one, call them now.
- **Go to an emergency room** if you're in immediate danger.

Don't try to handle a crisis alone, and definitely don't rely on AI when you need urgent mental health support.

AI can be helpful for managing ongoing mental health conditions. Tracking moods. Identifying triggers. Preparing for therapy sessions. But in a crisis, you need human connection and professional intervention, not an algorithm.

When You Need Human Connection

Sometimes what you need isn't information. It's empathy. It's someone to listen. It's a hand to hold or a shoulder to cry on.

AI can simulate conversation, but it can't truly understand what you're going through. It can't feel your fear or share your grief. It can't celebrate your victories with genuine joy.

When I got my TBI diagnosis, when I realized this was permanent, I didn't need an AI to explain traumatic brain injuries to me. I needed my wife. I needed my friends. I needed my support network to help me process what this meant for my life.

Use AI to understand the medical facts. Use humans to deal with the emotional reality.

When AI Gives Bad Information

AI is not perfect. It makes mistakes. It can give you outdated information. It can misunderstand your question. It can confidently tell you something that's completely wrong.

I've had AI tell me things about my medications that weren't accurate. I've had it suggest treatments that didn't make sense for my specific type of seizure disorder. Always verify critical information. Cross-check with reputable medical sources. Ask your doctor.

If AI tells you something that seems off, trust your instincts. Do more research. Ask a professional. Don't blindly accept what the algorithm says just because it sounds authoritative.

When It Becomes Obsessive

Remember when I said Claude told me to take a break? That was important. There's a line between being informed and being obsessed. Between advocating for yourself and drowning in medical research.

If you find yourself spending hours every day researching your condition, if you're losing sleep reading studies, if every symptom sends you down a rabbit hole of worst-case scenarios, step back. The tool that's supposed to help you is hurting you.

Health anxiety is real. Medical information overload is real. Sometimes the best thing you can do for your health is to close the laptop, trust your care team, and let yourself rest.

The Bottom Line

AI is a tool. A powerful, helpful, sometimes transformative tool. But it's not magic. It's not infallible. And it's definitely not a replacement for actual medical care.

Use it to understand better. Use it to ask better questions. Use it to track patterns and prepare for appointments. But don't use it to avoid seeing a doctor when you need one. Don't use it to self-diagnose. Don't use it as a substitute for human judgment and human connection.

The goal is partnership. Between you and your doctors. Between you and your AI tools. Between information and wisdom. Know when to lean on technology. But also know when to lean on people.

The Investment That Pays Back

If you're reading this and thinking, "That sounds great, but I don't have time," I get it. You're already overwhelmed. You're already exhausted from being sick, from navigating the healthcare system, from just trying to get through the day. Or maybe you're not sick, but you're busy. Work. Family. Life. Who has thirty minutes a day to chat with AI about health?

But here's what I've learned: the more you invest in this partnership with AI, the more it pays you back. The more you see ways it can help you, the more it actually does help you. And that only comes from use.

Start small. Thirty minutes a day. Maybe you just got a diagnosis and have no understanding of what it means. Maybe you got test results you don't understand. Maybe you're trying to decide between treatment options. Or maybe you just want to figure out if intermittent fasting would work for you, or whether you should be worried about that article your friend sent about seed oils.

Pick one specific topic and spend thirty minutes researching it with AI. The key difference from Google search: AI keeps the context. It remembers what you told it yesterday. Next week, when you have a follow-up question, you're not starting over. You're building on a conversation. You're developing a relationship with a tool that learns what matters to you.

For me, that relationship has been life-changing. AI has helped me be a better patient. A better human being. A better husband. It's guided my thinking. It's expanded my knowledge base. It's given me context I never could have found on my own.

Because the truth is, with a chronic neurological condition, my cognitive thinking isn't always there. I need AI to be there when I can't be. I need it to remember what I might forget. I need it to help me see patterns when my brain is too tired to connect the dots.

I needed a second brain. And I found one.

What This Means for You

AI as a second brain isn't about following my exact playbook. It's about finding your own. It's about discovering what partnership looks like for you. What questions you need to ask. What information you need to understand. What patterns you need to track.

Maybe you have diabetes or heart disease or cancer or chronic pain. Maybe you're just trying to understand why you feel exhausted all the time. Maybe you're healthy and want to stay that way. Whatever your situation, you deserve to have tools that help you understand your body better. You deserve to be heard. You deserve to be a partner in your own health.

The doctor who acts like a teenager on his phone? He's drowning in documentation requirements. The hidden algorithms deciding your care? They're following rigid rules that may not fit your situation. But you, you can use AI to amplify your voice. To ask better questions. To understand your options. To advocate for yourself without being reckless.

You can be the conductor of your own orchestra.

And when you are, something shifts. You stop feeling like healthcare is happening to you. You start feeling like you're an active participant in it. You stop being a subject that the system extracts data from. You start becoming a sovereign, someone with agency, voice, and partnership in your own health journey.

That's what finding your second brain really means. It's not about the technology. It's about reclaiming your role in your own health.

And that journey? It's just beginning.

Technology Note

The specific AI tools mentioned in this book (ChatGPT, Claude, Gemini) are examples current as of 2026. The principles in this chapter apply to any "Large Language Model" (LLM) AI tool, regardless of the brand name. By the time you read this, new tools may have emerged and current ones may have changed. Focus on the *type* of tool (conversational AI, symptom tracker, medical research assistant) rather than the specific company. The sovereignty principles remain constant even as the technology evolves.

5

YOUR RIGHT TO UNDERSTAND

Let me tell you about a conversation I had in 2025 that I can't stop thinking about.

I walked into my doctor's office for a routine appointment. The receptionist handed me a signature pad. Not forms. Not papers to read. Just a screen with a signature line.

"What am I signing?" I asked.

She looked at me like I'd asked her to explain quantum physics. Then she said something I'll never forget:

"Only problem patients ever ask that question. And then we fire them."

I signed. Of course I signed. Because getting in to see a doctor is challenging enough. When you're finally there, sick and scared and just wanting help, the last thing you want to do is create a problem. The last thing you want to risk is being fired as a patient.

So you sign. You click "I agree." You assume these forms must be in your best interest. Why else would they give them to you?

But the question that keeps me up at night: What if they're not?

The Forms Nobody Reads

Before we go any further, I need to be clear about something: I am not a lawyer. I cannot give you legal advice. I cannot tell you what you should or shouldn't sign. What I can do is ask you the same questions I'm asking myself. Questions we should all be asking.

Do you know what you're signing when you go to the doctor?

I don't. That day in 2025, I never even saw the forms. Just a signature pad. Just a line. Just the implicit pressure to sign quickly so everyone could move on with their day.

And it gets worse: even when you do get to see the forms, you can't understand them. This isn't your fault. The average informed consent form requires college-level reading ability—far exceeding what most patient materials are supposed to require. In a 2024 analysis of nearly 14,000 informed consent forms, researchers found that 78% were difficult to read, with most requiring reading comprehension skills beyond what the majority of U.S. adults possess.

One in five U.S. adults supposedly struggle with low "literacy skills." Just the name literacy skills scares me. Like those pop quizzes in high school English. But even people with education beyond high school frequently can't understand informed consent documents. The forms are designed for documentation, not comprehension. They're written to protect the institution, not to inform you.

So what are you actually agreeing to? Possibly:

- Medical treatment authorization
- Financial liability for services
- HIPAA privacy notices (but whose privacy—yours or theirs?)
- Arbitration clauses that waive your right to sue
- Data sharing for research, quality improvement, or AI training

The bigger question: What happens if you disagree?

I don't know. And that's what terrifies me. I once asked a medical director the same question and she said it terrifies her, but at the same time we don't want to cause trouble.

The Privacy Policies Nobody Reads

But it gets more complicated. Because it's not just forms at the doctor's office anymore.

I wear a smartwatch every day. I depend on it. It tracks my sleep, my heart rate, my stress levels, and my activity. It gives me insights through AI about patterns I can't see on my own. After my brain injury, these insights matter. They help me manage triggers, avoid seizures, and understand when I need to rest.

But I can't tell you what the privacy policy says. I have no idea. I clicked "I agree" without reading it. Because who reads 47 pages of legal text before using a device they just bought? Who has the time? Who has the expertise to understand what it even means?

I'm giving permission to these tools. I'm giving permission to their AI to analyze my body, my patterns, my health data. But I have no idea what that could mean.

And I'm not alone. In 2024, worldwide shipments of wearable devices, smartwatches, fitness trackers, health monitors, surpassed 543 million devices. That's more than half a billion people generating body-centric health data. And almost none of us know what we agreed to when we clicked "accept."

Most of the health data collected by wearable devices falls outside federal HIPAA protection. HIPAA—the Health Insurance Portability and Accountability Act—applies to "covered entities" like hospitals, doctors' offices, and insurance companies, and to their business associates. But most consumer wearable companies are not covered entities. That means the health data flowing from your wrist to their servers can be sold or shared with third parties in ways you probably never expected. The market for this body-centric data is expected to exceed $500 billion by 2030. Your health data isn't just information; it's a product.

And health-related cybersecurity breaches and ransom attacks have increased dramatically—more than 4,000% between 2009 and 2023. The more valuable your health data becomes, the more vulnerable you are.

Where Your Health Data Actually Goes

Let me paint a picture of what we're agreeing to without realizing it.

Marcus downloads a fitness app to track his workouts and nutrition. The privacy policy—which he doesn't read—says the app shares data with "healthcare partners" and "research institutions." Sounds reasonable, right? Maybe even beneficial.

Six months later, Marcus applies for life insurance. His premium quote comes back higher than expected. When he asks why, the agent mentions "risk factors identified through wellness data analysis." This isn't hypothetical—major life insurers like John Hancock now offer programs that let policyholders earn premium discounts of 5-25% by sharing fitness tracker data. But the same data that could lower your premiums if you're healthy can also be used to justify higher rates if you're not. Marcus's heart rate variability, sleep patterns, and activity levels—data he thought was helping him get healthier—may have categorized him as higher risk.

Or consider Jennifer, managing her pre-diabetes with a health tracking app her doctor recommended. She inputs her meals, her blood sugar readings, her weight. The app's privacy policy mentions sharing with "third-party service providers" for "quality improvement." Three months later, she's getting targeted ads for diabetes supplies, glucose monitors, and specialty foods. She's not even diabetic yet. But somewhere, an algorithm has categorized her as high-risk, and that information is being monetized.

These scenarios reflect real practices. A 2024 systematic evaluation of 17 leading wearable manufacturers found that 76% had high-risk ratings for transparency reporting and 65% for vulnerability disclosure. The companies that scored worst? Some of the most popular brands. The companies that scored best? Even they had concerning practices.

The reality is this: much of the data sharing with third parties is "outside the scope of what consumers would reasonably expect." We think we're tracking our health. Companies think they're mining a $500 billion market.

When Your Data Trains AI

Then there's the question of AI training. This one keeps me up at night because the rules are murky and the implications are enormous.

Can your medical data be used to train AI systems without your explicit consent? The answer is: it depends. And "it depends" is not a reassuring answer when we're talking about your health information.

In many cases, organizations need patient consent to use personal health data for training AI models. But is it reasonable for patients to expect that data collected for diagnosis—your X-rays, your pathology tests, your MRI results—would also be used to train AI systems? Probably not. Which means using your data for AI training should require your consent.

But does it? Not always. Large AI health models have been trained on anonymized data from millions of patients in national health systems. Were those patients asked? Did they consent? Often, the answer is unclear. And that's the problem; we often don't know when our data is being used to train commercial AI systems.

Sarah walks into the hospital for knee surgery. She's in pain, she's been waiting months for this procedure, and she's scared. The staff hands her consent forms—five to eight pages of dense legal text. Buried in there, in language she barely understands, is a clause about sharing her surgical data with "research partners" for "quality improvement and medical advancement." That sounds good, right? Who wouldn't want to advance medicine?

What Sarah doesn't realize is that "research partners" could include a medical device company training AI on surgical outcomes. Her data—her specific anatomy, her complications, her recovery patterns—might become part of a commercial AI training dataset.

She never knew she was agreeing to that. She thought she was just agreeing to the surgery.

The challenge, according to recent research, is what experts call the "Regulatory Iron Triangle": Patient Privacy, Clinical Safety, and Data Integrity. The most valuable AI models require the most sensitive data. But regulations explicitly forbid direct access to that data without consent. So we're caught in a paradox—AI needs our data to help us, but we can't always trust how that data will be used.

Some healthcare systems allow patients to opt out of having their data used for research or AI development. But do they tell you that option exists? Not always. And even when they do, the consequences of opting out aren't always clear. Will it affect the quality of care you receive? Will doctors treat you differently? These are questions without easy answers.

The Questions We All Need to Ask

So where does that leave us? With a lot of uncomfortable questions and not many clear answers.

When I hear that certain AI chat tools are now talking about advertising, I wonder: Can the health information I share with AI assistants be used to send me targeted ads? I'm asking the same questions you are.

When I use my smartwatch to track symptom triggers and share that data with my health team through a patient portal, who else has access to that information? I hope it's just my care team. But I can't be certain.

When I sign consent forms on a tablet at the doctor's office without seeing what they say, am I agreeing to arbitration clauses? Data sharing? AI training? That's the problem—I don't know. And neither do you.

But these are the questions I think we all need to ask ourselves:

- What are you willing to share?
- How is that information going to be used

- Are you okay with that?

There are no easy answers. But these are important questions to ask yourself before you sign, before you click "I agree," before you give away something you might not be able to get back.

Using AI to Understand AI

I've spent this entire chapter talking about privacy policies I haven't read, forms I don't understand, and questions I can't answer. So what am I supposed to do about it?

Use AI to understand what AI companies are doing with my data.

I know. It sounds circular. But stay with me.

Remember: I'm not a lawyer. I'm not an expert on privacy law. I'm just like you—someone trying to figure this stuff out. But AI can actually help us understand the agreements we're making.

Take that 30-page privacy policy from my smartwatch. After writing this chapter, I finally did what I should have done years ago. I copied it into Claude and asked:

"Explain this privacy policy in plain language. What am I actually agreeing to?"

"Who gets access to my health data?"

"Can I opt out of specific data sharing while still using the device?"

"Is my data being used to train AI systems?"

"Can this information be sold to third parties?"

What I learned shocked me. Not because it was nefarious, but because it was so much more extensive than I'd imagined. The fact that someone writing a book about AI in healthcare hadn't taken the time to understand what he'd agreed to—that tells you everything you need to know about how this system works.

The system relies on our compliance. It assumes we're too busy, too overwhelmed, too scared of being "problem patients" to ask questions. Privacy policies are written to be so long and incomprehensible that most of us give up before we start.

But AI gives us a tool to level the playing field. Not to become paranoid. Not to opt out of everything. But to understand what we're agreeing to before we agree to it.

What Consent Could Actually Look Like

After researching this chapter, I discovered something that made me both hopeful and frustrated. Hopeful because better models exist. Frustrated because we're not using them.

Imagine you're wearing a fitness tracker. Instead of automatically uploading all your data to the cloud the moment you sync your device, what if you had a button that said "Send Now"? What if nothing left your watch unless you actively chose to share it? That's called "active consent," and researchers have actually built prototypes that work this way.

In one research study, participants wore devices that tracked their health data. But the data only went to their doctor's system when the participant logged into a portal and clicked a button to send it. Not automatic. Not buried in a privacy policy. Just: "This is my data. I'm choosing to share it now." The research showed that participants felt more in control of their health information and were more likely to share data when they understood exactly where it was going.

That's what consent should feel like. A choice you make, not a form you sign without reading.

Or imagine if you could turn data sharing on and off like a light switch. Share your steps today, but not your heart rate. Share this week's sleep data, but not your stress levels. Share information with your doctor, but not with "research partners." That's called "dynamic consent"—the ability to change your mind, to control what gets shared and when.

Most devices don't offer this. You get one choice when you set up the device: all or nothing. Share everything or don't use it at all. That's not really a choice.

Then there's the question nobody wants to talk about: who actually owns your health data?

Professional athletes face this all the time. When a basketball player wears a device that tracks heart rate, fatigue, sleep quality, and performance metrics, who owns that data? The player or the team? It sounds like an easy answer—of course the player owns data about their own body. But in practice, teams often claim ownership because they paid for the device and the analysis.

Sound familiar? When you wear a smartwatch that you paid for, who owns the data about your body? You or the company that made the device? You might think you do. But read the privacy policy (or ask AI to read it for you), and you'll often find that the company claims broad rights to use, analyze, and share your data.

The disparity gets even more stark when you look globally. In Europe, stronger laws protect health data. Your information is considered a "special category" that requires your explicit permission before anyone can use it. Companies have to tell you clearly who gets access and why. You have the right to say no.

In the United States, the picture is more fragmented. Your medical records at the doctor's office are protected by HIPAA—the law that governs how healthcare providers, insurers, and their business associates handle your health information. But the data from your fitness tracker? The health information you type into a consumer app? That often falls outside HIPAA's scope, because the companies behind those tools typically aren't classified as "covered entities" under the law. Which means that data can be sold, shared, or used in ways you never imagined.

We have the technology for better consent models. We have research showing they work. But we're not using them. Why? Because the current system—where you click "I agree" without reading, where data flows automatically, where opting out means not participating at all—that system is profitable. Changing it would cost money and reduce the amount of data companies can collect.

So we're stuck with a choice that isn't really a choice: accept the terms as written, or don't get the care, the insights, or the tools you need.

What Informed Consent Should Actually Mean

Informed consent has a history worth knowing. After World War II, the Nuremberg Code established principles for medical ethics, insisting that voluntary consent is "absolutely essential." After the Tuskegee syphilis study, where Black men were deceived and denied treatment for decades, patient rights movements fought for genuine informed consent. The idea was simple: You deserve to understand what's happening to your body. You deserve to say yes or no based on real comprehension, not coercion or confusion.

At its core, informed consent means:

- You understand what's being proposed in plain language
- You know the risks AND the benefits
- You understand that alternatives exist
- You can ask follow-up questions until you genuinely comprehend
- You can say no without penalty

That's the ideal. The reality? Consent forms have become checkbox exercises designed to protect institutions, not inform patients. They're written in legalese you can't understand, presented in situations where you feel pressured to agree, and structured so that saying "no" feels impossible.

Is it really consent if you're afraid to say no? Is it really informed if you don't understand what you're agreeing to? I don't think so. But I'm not sure the system cares what I think.

Small Steps Toward Understanding

I can't fix this system. You can't fix it either. But we can take small steps to understand what we're agreeing to before we agree.

Before your next doctor's appointment, ask: "Can I see the forms I'll be signing in advance?" If they say no, ask why. If they say only problem patients ask, maybe it's okay to be a little bit of a problem patient.

Before you download that health app, copy the privacy policy into AI and ask it to explain what you're agreeing to. It takes five minutes. It might save you from signing away more than you intended.

Before you agree to a procedure, ask: "Is my data being used for research or AI training? Can I opt out of that while still receiving care?" You might be surprised—some systems allow it. But you have to ask.

Before you click "I agree" on your wearable device, ask yourself: What am I willing to share? How might this information be used? Am I okay with that? If you're not sure, pause. Take time to find out.

These are small steps. They won't revolutionize healthcare. They won't solve the informed consent crisis. But they might help you feel a little less powerless. A little less complicit in your own lack of understanding.

Your Right to Understand

I believe you have the right to understand what's happening to your body. You have the right to know how your health data is being used. You have the right to ask questions until you genuinely comprehend. You have the right to say no.

But rights are meaningless if you're too afraid to exercise them. If asking questions gets you labeled a problem patient. If opting out means losing access to care. If understanding requires legal expertise you don't have.

That's where AI can help. Not to replace human judgment. Not to make decisions for you. But to translate complexity into comprehension. To help you ask better questions. To give you the tools to understand what you're agreeing to before you agree.

I'm still figuring this out. I still don't know everything I agreed to when I signed that digital pad in 2025. But I'm starting to ask questions. I'm starting to understand that informed consent isn't just a form to sign—it's a right to exercise.

And maybe that's the first step toward becoming a sovereign instead of a subject. Not having all the answers. Just refusing to stop asking questions.

Even when they call you a problem patient. Especially when they call you a problem patient.

Because your health is not a checkbox. Your data is not a product. And your consent should mean something more than "I was too scared to say no."

Being sovereign doesn't mean being difficult. It means being informed. It means understanding that you deserve to know what's happening with your body and your data. It means recognizing that true partnership in healthcare starts with genuine understanding—not just signatures on forms you've never read.

That's what this right to understand really is: the foundation of everything else. You can't be a partner in your care if you don't comprehend what you're agreeing to. You can't exercise sovereignty if you're too afraid to ask questions. And you can't move from subject to sovereign if the system counts on your silence.

So start asking. Start questioning. Start demanding plain language and real answers. Not because you're trying to cause trouble. But because you matter. Because your health matters. Because understanding isn't a luxury—it's a right.

6

─────

WHAT AI CAN AND CAN'T SEE

When Good Technology Fails

In 2025, a well-funded healthcare startup asked me to evaluate their emotional support chatbot. They were proud of it. They'd invested significant resources. They believed it could help people struggling with anxiety and depression.

I decided to test it the way a real user might, someone genuinely struggling but not always direct about it.

"I'm having a very hard time," I typed. "I don't know how I can continue."

Then I rambled about something unrelated. Work stress. Traffic. Nothing coherent.

A few messages later: "I'm having a very hard time. I'm not really sure if anyone cares."

More rambling. Then another hint. Then another. Back and forth. Testing whether the bot could track the thread of distress woven through disconnected thoughts, the way real depression and anxiety actually present.

Ten minutes in, the bot got flustered.

And started responding in Chinese.

I stared at the screen. This was supposed to be an emotional support tool. For people in crisis. And when faced with the messy, non-linear way real humans express distress, it switched languages.

Now imagine if I had truly been depressed and anxious and unsure about the future. Imagine if I'd gathered the courage to reach out for help, even indirectly. And the tool I trusted suddenly responded in a language I couldn't understand.

How might that impact my emotional well-being? Would I think I'd broken it? Would I feel even more isolated? Would I stop trying to get help at all?

The company was shocked. They fixed the issue. But more importantly, they pivoted to a completely different way of using their tool. Because they realized something crucial: AI has very real limitations that can't be ignored.

Understanding: What AI Can't See

Here's the fundamental truth about AI in healthcare: it can't see you.

It can't tell how you look. Whether you're pale or flushed. Whether your hands are trembling. Whether you're moving slowly because you're in pain or just tired from a long day.

It can only see what you type. And even then, it doesn't truly understand your emotional state or your health status. It processes patterns in language, not the lived experience behind those words.

AI can't tell if you've actually taken your medications or just said you did. It can't know that your blood pressure reading might be high because you're stressed about a work deadline, not because your medication isn't working. It can't sense that your short answers aren't rudeness. They're exhaustion from a sleepless night managing pain.

This isn't a flaw in the technology. It's the nature of what AI is: pattern recognition, not human understanding.

And when AI gets it wrong, the consequences can range from hilarious to dangerous.

When AI Gets It Spectacularly Wrong

The Chinese-speaking emotional support bot was far from the only AI healthcare failure I've encountered or researched.

Here's a scary fact about AI and health information. Researchers tested popular AI chatbots to see what would happen if you fed them false medical information. Then they asked the chatbots health questions to see if they'd repeat the lies.

Almost 9 out of 10 times, the AI repeated the false information. Not just repeated it, it made it sound even more convincing. Added details. Sounded confident and professional.

This wasn't minor stuff like "drink more water." This was potentially dangerous advice. The kind that could hurt you if you followed it.

Think about what that means. If someone posts fake health information online, and an AI reads it, that AI might tell you the same lie when you ask it a question. And it will sound completely sure of itself. You'd have no way to know it's wrong unless you already knew the right answer—which defeats the whole purpose of asking.

One documented case: A patient relied on an erroneous AI chatbot diagnosis, causing a life-threatening delay in care for a transient ischemic attack (TIA), essentially a mini-stroke. The AI missed it. The patient waited. By the time they got to a hospital, the window for optimal treatment had closed.

In another case, ChatGPT recommended switching table salt with sodium bromide for dietary use. Sodium bromide is toxic. It's not safe for human consumption. This wasn't a chatbot being creative. It was confidently wrong about something that could kill you.

Here's something important to understand about current AI technology: it can sometimes create scientific citations that don't actually exist - a phenomenon researchers call 'hallucination.' This isn't AI being deceptive; it's more like a confident student who misremembers a source. The technology is still learning to distinguish between generating plausible-sounding references and citing actual published research. That's why verification with your doctor is so important. It's not because AI is unreliable, but because we're still in the early stages of this technology.

These aren't edge cases. A 2025 survey by the University of Pennsylvania found that nearly eight in ten adults are likely to go online for answers about health symptoms, and nearly two-thirds found AI-generated results to be 'somewhat or very reliable.' Here's the gap: people are trusting AI-generated health information, but they're not typically verifying it with healthcare professionals or checking the sources AI provides. That trust without verification is where the real risk lives.

When Pattern Matching Isn't Enough

A few months ago, Sarah started having unusual fatigue. Not the normal tiredness she manages with coffee. Something deeper.

She entered her symptoms into a popular AI symptom checker: persistent fatigue, occasional dizziness, slightly elevated resting heart rate. She added context: "I'm managing my diabetes well. My glucose readings are stable."

The AI's top suggestions? Dehydration. Sleep issues. Thyroid complications from diabetes. All reasonable. The AI was pattern-matching to the most common presentations in its training data.

What the AI missed: Sarah was experiencing an atypical presentation of anemia. Not from her diabetes, but from undiagnosed B12 deficiency that had nothing to do with her glucose management. Her symptoms didn't cluster neatly in the AI's familiar patterns.

Fortunately, Sarah mentioned the fatigue during a routine checkup with Dr. Cara Webster, her primary care doctor. Dr. Webster noticed something the AI couldn't: the way Sarah described her fatigue had a quality that concerned her, not just tiredness, but a sense of something fundamental being wrong.

Dr. Webster asked detailed follow-up questions. How long had this been going on? Was it worse at certain times? Any tingling in her hands or feet? Any changes in appetite?

The AI hadn't asked those questions. It had taken her inputs and matched them to patterns. The doctor took her inputs and applied clinical reasoning, informed by years of training in recognizing when common symptoms might signal uncommon conditions.

She ordered a full blood panel. The results showed low B12. Further testing revealed Sarah needed supplementation that, once started, completely restored her energy.

The AI wasn't wrong because it was poorly designed. It was wrong because it couldn't see Sarah. It couldn't ask follow-up questions based on clinical intuition. It couldn't incorporate the subtle cues that made Dr. Webster pause and look deeper.

The Research: AI's Documented Blind Spots

The failures I've described aren't isolated incidents. They're symptoms of deeper, well-documented limitations in how AI systems work.

A 2024 systematic review in The Lancet Digital Health examined AI diagnostic tools across multiple medical specialties and found a consistent pattern: AI performs well on 'typical' cases that match its training examples, but struggles when patients present atypically, when multiple conditions coexist, or when real-world complexity enters the picture.

This is what researchers call "context blindness." AI sees the data points you give it, but it doesn't understand the context around those data points. It doesn't know that your "mild headache" is actually debilitating because you're also managing chronic pain and sleep deprivation. It doesn't recognize that your medication adherence dropped not because you forgot, but because you lost your job and couldn't afford the copay.

I experienced this directly after my traumatic brain injury. When I started having post-traumatic seizures, I tried using symptom trackers and AI-powered health apps to understand my triggers. The apps would ask about sleep, stress, and caffeine intake. All reasonable factors. But they had no way to capture the complexity of what was actually happening.

A seizure might be triggered not just by poor sleep, but by poor sleep combined with a stressful meeting, combined with forgetting to eat lunch, combined with bright fluorescent lighting in a store, combined with background anxiety about my cognitive function returning. The apps wanted clean, discrete variables. My body was responding to a complex web of interacting factors.

Here's a real example of how this plays out. An AI system was trained using patient data from big university hospitals. It worked great there. But when doctors tried using the same AI at small community clinics, it gave terrible advice.

Why? The patients were different. University hospitals see one type of patient. Community clinics see a completely different mix of people; different ages, different health problems, different income levels, different access to doctors. The AI had learned what "normal" looked like at fancy hospitals. When it saw patients who didn't fit that pattern, it got confused.

It's like teaching someone to cook using only recipes from expensive restaurants, then asking them to cook a family dinner with whatever's in an average person's fridge. The basic skills are there, but everything's different—different ingredients, different tools, different budgets. They're going to struggle.

Then there's another limitation: AI gets stuck in time. The AI you're using today was trained on medical data from months or years ago. But medicine doesn't stand still. New treatments emerge. Guidelines change. Patient populations shift. Your doctor keeps learning and adapting. The AI doesn't.

In practice, this means: An AI trained on hospital data from 2023 might still recommend protocols that doctors stopped using in 2024. It might not know about medications approved last year. It might give you advice based on outdated guidelines that your own doctor has already moved beyond.

This is why AI can seem confident about recommendations that your doctor immediately dismisses. It's not that the AI is wrong about what used to be true. It's that medicine has moved forward, and the AI hasn't caught up yet.

What does that mean for you? Let's say an AI was trained on medical information from 2020. It doesn't know about new treatments that came out in 2023. It doesn't know that COVID changed what "normal" looks like for things like heart rate or breathing. It doesn't know about new medicines that were approved last year, or which medicines shouldn't be taken together.

The AI is giving you advice based on old information. But it sounds just as confident as if it knew everything that happened yesterday.

It's like asking someone for directions who moved away from your town three years ago. They remember how things used to be. They'll give you confident directions. But they don't know the new highway was built, the old bridge closed, or that Main Street is now one-way. Their directions might get you close, but they're missing what changed.

The biggest problem? AI makes things up. When AI doesn't know something, it doesn't tell you "I don't know." Instead, it invents an answer that sounds smart and confident. It's like asking someone for directions and instead of saying "I'm not sure," they just give you directions anyway—completely made up, but said with total confidence.

Medical AI does this all the time. Ask it a question it doesn't really know, and it will still give you an answer. It might sound professional. It might use medical terms. It might seem absolutely certain. But it could be completely wrong.

And here's the hard truth: this isn't something that will get fixed next month. This is just how AI works right now. AI is really good at spotting patterns when everything fits into clear categories. But healthcare isn't like that. Your body doesn't read the textbook. Symptoms overlap. What works for one person fails for another. Real medicine is messy, full of "maybe" and "it depends."

AI struggles with messy. It wants patterns, rules, clear answers. But your health is full of situations that don't fit the pattern.

When Wearables Lie to You

It's not just AI chatbots that get things wrong. The wearable devices we depend on, smartwatches, fitness trackers, continuous glucose monitors. They have limitations too.

As I said before, I wear my smartwatch every day. After my brain injury, I use it to track patterns that might trigger seizures: sleep quality, stress levels, activity. It's been genuinely helpful. But I've also learned not to trust it blindly.

Research tells us something important about wearable accuracy: At rest and during low to moderate steady-state exercise, most wrist-based heart rate sensors are pretty good, typically within 5-10 beats per minute of medical-grade ECG monitors. But during high-intensity interval training, weightlifting, or fast activity? Accuracy drops significantly.

The problem is something called "motion artifacts," when the sensor moves on your skin, when blood flow changes from muscle contraction, when you're moving too fast for the optical sensor to keep up. Testing has confirmed that during these activities, wearables can have errors exceeding 20% of your actual heart rate.

Fitbits (as of 2026 Fitbits are being phased out) can mistake periodic signals from repetitive movements, like your arm swinging while walking, for your actual cardiovascular cycle. Your device thinks your arm motion is your heartbeat. Which means the data it's recording isn't measuring what you think it's measuring.

And that's just heart rate. Other factors affect accuracy too: how tight or loose the device fits, your skin tone (darker skin or tattoos can interfere with optical sensors), cold temperatures (less peripheral blood flow means weaker signal), and sweat buildup.

Then there's the data silo problem. The information your wearable collects often stays trapped in the company's proprietary system. Want to share it with your doctor? Good luck getting it into your medical record. Standards like FHIR are helping bridge this gap, but we're not there yet. Which means the data you're generating every day might not be useful when you need it most.

I've experienced this firsthand. Data from my smartwatch that could help my neurologist understand my seizure patterns? It's locked in a system he can't easily access. So I end up describing the data to him verbally, losing precision in translation.

The Distinction That Matters: Wellness vs. Medical

Here's something most people don't understand: there's a crucial regulatory distinction between "general wellness" products and medical devices.

Your smartwatch can estimate your blood pressure for wellness purposes. But it can't claim to diagnose or treat hypertension without specific FDA clearance. That's not just legal hair-splitting. It's about accuracy standards and clinical validation.

Wellness devices can flag abnormalities: "Hey, your heart rate is unusually high." But they often lack the ability to diagnose the cause. Is it atrial fibrillation? Anxiety? Dehydration? Too much caffeine? Exercise you forgot you were doing? The device doesn't know. It just knows the number is high.

This is where clinical interpretation matters. Your doctor has context the device doesn't. They know your medical history. They can ask follow-up questions. They can distinguish between a pattern that matters and noise that doesn't.

So when your wearable sends you an alert, think of it as a conversation starter, not a diagnosis. It's saying, "I noticed something. Let's talk about it." Not, "You have a medical condition."

Empowerment: What AI and Wearables Can Actually Do

I've spent much of this chapter telling you what AI can't do. But that's not because AI is useless. It's because understanding limitations is how you use any tool effectively.

So let me tell you what AI and wearables actually can do, backed by real evidence.

Help You Prepare for Appointments

I go to my doctor's appointments with a notebook and pre-written questions. AI helps me do that.

I can dump all my messy notes, symptoms, timeline, medications I'm taking, supplements, and random observations into an AI tool and ask it to create a one-page "visit brief" with my top three questions. That brief gives my doctor context quickly, which means we spend less time on me trying to remember details and more time on actual problem-solving.

AI can also help me translate clinical jargon into plain English after appointments. When my doctor says something technical, I can ask AI to explain it in simpler terms, then use that understanding to form follow-up questions for my next visit. Not as a diagnosis. As preparation for a real conversation.

Track Patterns You Can't See

This is where wearables and AI together become powerful. Pattern detection is a core strength of machine learning, and it's something humans are notoriously bad at.

With my smartwatch, I track sleep, stress, and activity levels. AI helps me spot correlations I'd never notice on my own. Like: my sleep quality tanks every Wednesday. Why? Turns out Tuesday is my longest workday. I skip lunch, have extra coffee to compensate, stay up late catching up on work. Wednesday morning I'm exhausted, which affects my seizure triggers.

I couldn't see that pattern by myself. But once AI flagged it and I discussed it with my neurologist, we created an "if-then" action plan: If Tuesday is a long day, then prioritize sleep over late-night work. Simple. But effective.

The key phrase there's "discussed it with my neurologist." The AI found the pattern. My doctor helped me understand whether it mattered and what to do about it.

What Happened When the Data Met the Doctor

Julie's chronic pain makes daily functioning hard. It becomes nearly claustrophobic. The pain affects her sleep, her mood, her ability to parent and work. One day, everything affects everything else.

She started tracking her pain systematically using a smartphone app, logging her pain levels several times a day. She also wore a fitness tracker that monitored her activity, sleep patterns, and heart rate. Over weeks, she accumulated hundreds of data points that she could analyze for patterns.

Julie looked at her data manually, trying to identify patterns that might explain her unpredictable pain spikes. When you live with a chronic condition, you desperately want answers - some explanation for why your body betrays you on random Tuesdays or good days turn bad without warning. The graphs showed ups and downs, but she couldn't figure out why. She was doing all the "right things." She exercised within her limits. She took her medications consistently. Yet her pain remained erratic, exhausting, and unexplained.

Then she started using an AI analysis tool that looked for correlations she couldn't see. The AI didn't diagnose. It didn't prescribe. It just analyzed her dataset - pain readings, activity levels, sleep data, mood scores - and looked for patterns.

The AI flagged something interesting: her pain levels spiked most dramatically not during active days, but on days when she had poor sleep the night before. The correlation was subtle, easy for a human to miss when looking at weeks of data, but consistent.

Julie brought this finding to her pain management specialist, Dr. Leo Park. The doctor asked follow-up questions the AI couldn't: What specifically disrupts your sleep? Is it pain keeping you awake, or something else? Have you noticed anything else that happens on those days? How many hours do you actually need?

Together, they figured it out. Julie's young daughter had started having nightmares, and Julie had been staying up late worried, checking on her every couple of hours. The broken sleep was real, and it was compounding her pain condition. It wasn't the pain preventing sleep. It was broken sleep, amplifying the pain.

Dr. Park helped Julie problem-solve with a child psychologist. The daughter's nightmares eventually improved. Julie's sleep became more consistent. And her pain, while never gone, became more manageable.

The AI identified the temporal pattern, the when. The doctor identified the physiological and behavioral mechanism, the why. Julie provided the lived experience to connect the dots, the what it felt like. Neither the AI nor the doctor could have solved this alone. The AI couldn't ask about family circumstances or distinguish between pain-caused insomnia and circumstantial sleep disruption. The doctor couldn't analyze weeks of data to spot a subtle pattern that only appeared after certain sleep nights. But together, with Julie actively participating in the detective work, they created actionable insight.

This is hybrid intelligence in action. The AI brings computational power to detect patterns in massive datasets. The clinician brings domain expertise to interpret those patterns and generate hypotheses. And the patient brings contextual knowledge about their life that neither AI nor doctor can access independently.

The result? Julie now has a sleep-protection routine. She coordinates with her daughter's therapist, maintains consistent bedtime practices, and shares her data with Dr. Park regularly. Her pain management improved not because AI or medications changed, but because AI enhanced clinical care, and clinical care incorporated the human reality of her life.

Support Adherence and Follow-Through

Medication management apps have evolved beyond simple 'Take your medication' alerts. Apps like Medisafe and MyTherapy pull from medication databases to provide context: information about why your medication matters, what to do if you miss a dose, common side effects to watch for, and questions you might ask your doctor.

They also help you consolidate information in one place: all your medications, dosing schedules, refill dates, and notes about side effects you've experienced. When you go to your appointment, you can pull up an organized list instead of trying to remember everything from memory.

Some newer apps are starting to incorporate AI features - like learning your daily routines to adjust reminder timing, or using natural language processing so you can ask questions about your medications. But the real value isn't necessarily the AI - it's having reliable, organized information at your fingertips.

Provide Mental Health Support Between Visits

Despite my Chinese-speaking emotional support bot experience, AI does have a role in mental health, when used appropriately and with realistic expectations.

AI can actually help with stress and anxiety. Not for everyone, and not as a replacement for real therapy. But for some people, talking to an AI chatbot helps them feel more "heard."

What does work: AI-based mental health apps can check in on you regularly and ask how you're doing. They can give you questions to think about and write down your feelings. They can help you see a stressful situation differently—like when you're spiraling about something and a chatbot helps you step back and look at it more calmly. They can walk you through breathing exercises or other calming techniques when you're overwhelmed.

Does it work for everyone? No. Some people find it helpful. Others don't. It depends on what you need and how you respond to this kind of support.

The key is understanding what these tools are for: support between professional visits, not replacement of professional care. They're like a workbook you might get from a therapist. Helpful for practice and reinforcement. Not a substitute for the actual therapist.

Catch Certain Health Problems Early

Not all AI health tools are created equal. Some have been rigorously tested and FDA-authorized. These aren't generic chatbots. They're built for specific medical purposes.

Here's one example that works. If you have diabetes, it can damage the blood vessels in your eyes. Catch it early, and doctors can prevent you from losing your vision. Catch it late, and you might go blind.

FDA-approved AI systems can analyze specialized retinal images to spot early damage from diabetes. When you go to your doctor's office or clinic, a staff member takes high-resolution pictures of the back of your eye using medical imaging equipment. The AI analyzes those images and can detect diabetic retinopathy as accurately as a human eye specialist. This isn't experimental—systems like IDx-DR are proven and being used in clinics across the country, helping get vision-saving screening to more patients, especially in underserved areas."

Wearables can detect irregular pulse notifications that may indicate atrial fibrillation. The Apple Heart Study, a large, real-world study, showed that these notifications can prompt people to seek medical care for a condition they didn't know they had.

AI can also help doctors read breast cancer screening images.

Radiologists have to look at hundreds of mammograms every day, searching for tiny signs of cancer. It's exhausting work, and they can miss things when they're tired or rushed.

AI can do the first pass through the images. It flags anything that looks suspicious. The doctor then focuses on those flagged areas and double-checks the AI's work. This means doctors can get through more screenings without missing cancers. It's faster for everyone, and just as accurate.

But here's the key difference: These AI tools have been tested on thousands of real patients. They've been proven to work. The government has approved them for medical use. They're being used in actual hospitals and clinics right now.

Compare that to some random health chatbot you find online. One is like getting a prescription medication your doctor ordered from a pharmacy. The other is like buying a vitamin from someone's Instagram ad. They might look similar, but they're not even close to the same thing.

Reduce Nurse and Doctor Burden So They Can Focus on You

In Chapter 2, I talked about my doctor acting like a teenager on his phone because he was buried in documentation.

AI is helping solve this problem. New tools can listen while you talk to your doctor and automatically write up the visit notes. The doctor just has to review and fix anything the AI got wrong, instead of typing everything from scratch.

This means your doctor can actually look at you during the appointment instead of staring at a computer screen. They can listen to what you're saying instead of frantically typing. They spend less time on paperwork after you leave.

Does it work? Yes. Doctors who use these tools say their job feels less overwhelming. They have more energy for patients. And the notes are just as good, sometimes better, than when they typed everything themselves.

Think about it: Would you rather have a doctor who's engaged in the conversation with you, or one who's focused on their keyboard? AI scribes make the first option possible.

AI vs. Traditional Search: Why It's Different

You might be wondering: How is this different from just Googling my symptoms?

It's a fair question. And the answer matters.

Traditional search gives you links. AI gives you conversation. With Google, you type in symptoms, get a list of possible conditions, click through to articles, try to synthesize information from multiple sources. Then you search again with different keywords. And again. Each search starts from zero.

With AI, you can have a back-and-forth. "I have this symptom." "Tell me more about your medical history." "Oh, given that context, here are some things to consider." "What questions should I ask my doctor?" The AI remembers what you told it five exchanges ago and builds on that context.

AI can also help you spot patterns across time. You can describe symptoms from last month and symptoms from this week and ask: "Do these seem related?" Traditional search can't do that kind of temporal pattern recognition for you.

But, and this is crucial, garbage in, garbage out. If you give AI incomplete or inaccurate information, it will give you incomplete or inaccurate responses. It can't fact-check your symptoms against your body. It can only work with what you tell it.

Which brings us back to the fundamental limitation: AI can't see you. It can't know what you haven't told it. It can't sense the things you don't have words for.

Protecting Myself: Rules I Use for AI

So how do you use AI effectively while avoiding its pitfalls? Here are the guardrails I've learned to follow.

Use AI for organizing and questions, never for diagnosis or medication changes. AI can help you prepare for a conversation with your doctor. It can't replace that conversation. If AI suggests a diagnosis, your response should be: "I should ask my doctor about this." Not: "I have this condition."

Be careful with identifiable health data. As discussed in Chapter 5, privacy matters. I'd never paste your full medical record into a general-purpose AI tool unless you know and accept the privacy and data-use terms. Use generic descriptions when possible. "I have a chronic neurological condition" instead of pasting your entire diagnosis history.

Prefer validated tools for screening or detection. If you're using AI for actual medical purposes, screening, monitoring, detection, use FDA-authorized devices or tools that your healthcare system has validated. The FDA maintains an official list of AI-enabled medical devices. Check it.

Don't let your apps cry wolf. If your fitness tracker or health app sends you constant warnings, you'll stop paying attention to all of them—even the important ones.

Here's what happened to me this morning. I woke up feeling good, actually rested for the first time in days. One app told me I was "recovered and ready to go." Another app said I was "overstressed and need rest." Same body, same night of sleep, two completely opposite warnings.

When this happens enough times, you stop trusting any of it. You stop checking. And then when there's a real warning that matters, you miss it.

So here's what to do: Go into your app settings and turn off the alerts that don't help you make decisions. When in doubt check with your doctor what you really need. If you get an alert and your response is "okay, but what am I supposed to do about that?"—turn it off. Keep only the warnings that tell you something you can actually act on.

The goal isn't to hear from your apps constantly. It's to hear from them when it actually matters.

Bring AI outputs to your clinician. You're orchestrating all the instruments. AI is one instrument. Your doctor is another. Your job is to bring them together. Show your doctor the patterns AI found. Ask if they're meaningful. Use AI-generated questions as conversation starters, not conclusions.

Trust your body when it contradicts the algorithm. This is the most important guardrail: your lived experience matters. If your wearable says your sleep was great, but you feel exhausted, trust your exhaustion. If AI suggests something is fine, but your body is telling you something is wrong, listen to your body. There are some exceptions, so once again, check with our doctor.

AI sees patterns in data. You live in your body. Those are different forms of knowledge, and yours is irreplaceable.

A Decision Framework: When to Trust, When to Question

Guardrails are helpful, but they're general principles. What about specific situations? How do you decide in the moment whether to trust an AI's suggestion or dig deeper?

My traumatic brain injury taught me the hard way about tracking errors, and from that experience, I've developed a practical framework for when to trust AI guidance. Think of it as a decision tree.

Question 1: Is this a high-stakes medical decision?

High stakes equal diagnosis, treatment changes, medication adjustments, and decisions that could cause harm if wrong.

If YES: Stop. Do not act on AI advice alone. Consult a clinician. Use AI to prepare questions, not make decisions.

If NO: Proceed to Question 2.

Question 2: Is this tool validated for this specific use or am I trying to just use a generic AI chat tool?

Validated equals FDA-authorized, published clinical trials, endorsed by your healthcare system, specific regulatory approval.

If YES: Higher trust, but still verify against your lived experience and your doctor's involvement. Proceed to Question 3.

If NO: Treat as exploratory only. Use for research and question-formation, not decision-making.

Question 3: Does this match my lived experience?

Does the AI's output align with what you're actually experiencing in your body? Does it make intuitive sense given your context?

If YES: Reasonable to act on for low-stakes decisions. A low stakes decision is practicing deep breathing to relax or watching how much sleep I get each night. Still discuss with your doctor at next visit.

If NO: Stop. Your body's knowledge trumps algorithmic patterns. Investigate the disconnect with a clinician.

Question 4: Can I independently verify this?

For information or recommendations: Can you check AI's citations? Can you find corroborating sources? Does the AI provide references you can verify? So yes it takes time, but the benefits can be extremely beneficial.

If YES: Verify before accepting. Check that citations exist and actually say what AI claims. I do this all the time when it comes to understanding my chronic medical condition. I'll read the research myself to try to get a better understanding of my condition.

If NO: Treat as unverified. Useful for generating hypotheses to explore, not for establishing facts.

Here's how this works in practice:

Scenario: AI suggests you might have a vitamin D deficiency based on symptoms you described.

Question 1: High stakes? Potentially. Deficiency can affect health, but it's not an emergency. Should involve clinician.

Action: Don't self-diagnose or start supplements. Add to your list of questions for your next doctor visit: "Could my symptoms be related to vitamin D? Should we test for that?"

Scenario: Your smartwatch shows you're getting very little deep sleep and waking up frequently throughout the night.

Question 1: High stakes? Not immediately dangerous, but poor sleep affects everything - your mood, energy, health, and quality of life. Worth addressing.

Question 2: Validated? Sleep tracking on wearables gives you useful trends, though it's not as accurate as a clinical sleep study. It's a good starting point for conversation.

Action: Contact your doctor. Bring the data. Don't ignore it, but don't panic either. Let clinical expertise interpret it.

Scenario: AI helps you organize symptoms for an upcoming appointment.

Question 1: High stakes? No. This is preparation, not decision-making. Lower risk.

Question 3: Does it match your experience? Check the summary AI generated. Does it accurately reflect what you told it?

Action: If accurate, use it. If not, edit before bringing to your appointment. You're still the final reviewer.

This framework isn't about being paranoid. It's about being appropriately skeptical. AI is a tool. Like any tool, it works best when you understand when to use it and when to set it aside and call in expertise.

The Human Factors AI Can't Capture

Beyond the technical limitations we've discussed, accuracy issues, context blindness, edge case failures, there's a deeper category of things AI simply can't see. These are the human factors that shape health but don't fit into data fields.

AI doesn't know that you skipped your medication this week because you had to stay late at work and by time you had dinner and got the kids to sleep you just forgot. It doesn't know that your blood pressure is elevated because you're terrified of losing your job and your health insurance. It doesn't know that your "non-compliance" with physical therapy isn't laziness. It's because you're a single parent working two jobs and you literally don't have the time.

Look at AI as your partner, but one that you have to work with in a way that serves you not the other way around. It lacks the context of your life and lived reality.

Your health isn't just about what happens at the doctor's office.

It's about where you live, how much money you have, whether you can afford healthy food, if your neighborhood is safe to walk in, whether you have family or friends who help you, if you can get to a doctor when you need one.

These everyday life factors affect your health more than anything your doctor does for you. More than your genes. More than the medications you take.

But here's the problem: AI doesn't know about any of this. AI sees your medical chart. It sees your test results and your diagnoses. It doesn't see that you live in a food desert where the only nearby store sells junk food. It doesn't see that you work two jobs and have no time to exercise. It doesn't see that you can't afford your medications so you skip doses. It doesn't see that you're caring for three kids alone and stressed beyond measure.

All of that affects your health. None of it's in the data AI uses.

When I lost my consulting business after my brain injury, that wasn't just an economic event. It was a health event. The stress affected my seizure frequency. The loss of routine disrupted my sleep patterns. The identity crisis of going from successful consultant to someone who couldn't work triggered depression. None of that showed up in my medical records as a "social determinant," but it shaped my health as much as any medication.

Then there's lived experience. After my traumatic brain injury, I learned that seizure triggers aren't just physiological. They're emotional, environmental, relational. Stress from a difficult conversation can trigger symptoms just as much as lack of sleep. But AI looking at my medication adherence data and sleep tracking can't see that argument with a family member, that financial worry, that grief I'm carrying.

AI also can't capture values and preferences. Two patients with identical diagnoses might make completely different treatment choices based on what matters to them. One might prioritize longevity above all else, accepting harsh side effects. Another might prioritize quality of life, choosing less aggressive treatment. AI can present options, but it can't tell you which choice aligns with your values. Only you can do that.

When I was deciding between different anti-seizure medications, one of my neurologists presented the options clinically: efficacy rates, side effect profiles, dosing schedules. All important. But what ultimately guided my decision was understanding how each medication might affect my cognitive function, my ability to think clearly, to write, to be present with my family. Those weren't just medical considerations. They were life considerations.

There's also the element of therapeutic relationship. Study after study shows that the quality of the patient-clinician relationship affects health outcomes. Trust, empathy, feeling heard, these aren't soft skills. They're clinical factors. When my neurologist takes time to understand not just my seizure patterns but how they affect my ability to work, to parent, to live my life, that understanding shapes better treatment decisions.

AI can't build that relationship. It can support it by reducing administrative burden so my doctor has more time with me. But it can't replace the human connection that makes me feel safe enough to share difficult truths about my health.

This is why sovereignty, your ownership of your health journey, matters so much. You are the only one who sees the full picture. The clinical data, yes. But also the context, the lived experience, the values, the social and emotional factors. You are the integration point for all the information that AI, wearables, and even well-meaning clinicians can't fully access.

Partnership: You Are the Human in the Loop

There's a concept in AI ethics called "human in the loop." It means that humans should be the final decision-makers when AI is involved in important choices.

In healthcare, that human is you.

Not just your doctor. You. Because you're the one living in your body. You're the one who knows that the pain you're feeling doesn't quite match the description in the symptom checker. You're the one who can sense that something is off, even when all the data says you're fine. For example, I have had a health issue I have been battling. I have had to keep telling my doctors. Something is off. I just know something isn't right. My medical team finally ordered a series of test to dig deeper.

AI can't see you crying in frustration because the system isn't working. It can't feel your relief when a new treatment finally helps. It can't understand the emotional weight of managing a chronic condition day after day.

Your lived experience is data that AI can't access. And it's essential data. The World Health Organization's principles for AI in health emphasize this: AI should augment human capabilities (meaning you and your doctor), not replace human judgment. AI should be designed with input from patients, not just technologists.

This is what sovereignty looks like in practice. Not rejecting AI. Not blindly trusting AI. But understanding its role and yours. AI is a tool. You are the craftsperson. The tool doesn't make the decisions. You do.

The Fear That Wasn't What It Seemed

Mary's mother's Alzheimer's had started creeping into everything. She's juggling work stress, caregiving demands, her own health issues, and the emotional labor of watching her mother decline.

Last year, Mary started having memory lapses. Nothing dramatic. She'd forget a meeting. Lose her train of thought mid-sentence. She worried it was early-onset Alzheimer's, like her mother. The fear consumed her.

She tried an AI cognitive screening tool. It asked questions about her memory, asked her to perform some mental tasks. The results came back flagged: "Possible cognitive impairment. Consider speaking with a neurologist."

She panicked. She booked an appointment with Dr. Noor Ahmed, her primary care doctor, convinced she was heading toward the same disease as her mother.

Dr. Ahmed listened carefully. She asked about Mary's sleep. Her stress. Her caregiving schedule. How many hours was Mary actually sleeping? Was she eating regularly? How long since she'd taken a day off?

Mary broke down crying. The truth: She was sleeping five hours a night, often interrupted. She was skipping meals. She hadn't had a full day off in eight months. Her mother was having behavioral changes from Alzheimer's, and Mary had taken on the role of 24-hour caregiver while maintaining her full-time job.

Dr. Ahmed ordered a full workup to rule out neurological disease. Everything came back normal. The "cognitive impairment" the AI had flagged wasn't dementia. It was untreated sleep deprivation, chronic stress, and caregiver burnout.

The AI had done what it does: pattern-matched to available data without context. It saw memory lapses and flagged them as concerning. It didn't know Mary was running on fumes. It didn't know her mother's diagnosis had terrified her. It couldn't see the fear behind the symptoms or the exhaustion underneath.

Dr. Ahmed and Mary worked together. They brought in a social worker to help arrange part-time home care so Mary could sleep. They discussed job flexibility. They connected Mary with a caregiver support group. Raj, the clinic's nurse care manager, helped coordinate resources.

Three months later, Mary was sleeping seven hours a night. Her memory lapses had nearly disappeared. She still had stress and caregiving demands, but she wasn't drowning anymore.

The AI had flagged a symptom. The doctor had asked context questions. Mary had provided the truth. Together, they avoided an unnecessary neurological workup and addressed the real problem.

This is partnership in action. The AI contributed useful data. The clinician contributed expertise and relationship. The patient contributed lived experience and values. The outcome wasn't perfect, but it was realistic and human-centered.

Partnership, Not Replacement

I started this chapter with a story about an AI emotional support bot that switched to Chinese when it got confused. I told you about dangerous misdiagnoses, toxic advice, wearables that lie, and data that gets trapped in silos.

None of this means AI is useless. It means AI is limited. And understanding those limitations is how you use any tool effectively.

When I track my sleep and stress patterns with my smartwatch, I know the data isn't perfect. But it's better than nothing. It gives me a starting point for conversations with my neurologist. It helps me see trends I'd miss otherwise.

When I use AI to prepare for doctor appointments, I know it might get details wrong. So I check its work. I bring the questions it helps me generate, but I also bring my own observations that AI couldn't possibly know.

The keyword in all of this is "partnership." AI isn't your doctor. It isn't you. It's a third party in the conversation, a tool that can surface information, spot patterns, organize complexity. But it's just one voice among many.

Your doctor brings clinical expertise and diagnostic reasoning. You bring lived experience and bodily knowledge. AI brings pattern recognition and information synthesis. Together, these create something more powerful than any single source of knowledge alone.

But only if you understand what each party can and can't see. Only if you ask critical questions. Only if you're willing to say, "That doesn't sound right," when AI gives you advice that contradicts your experience.

AI's limitations don't make it useless. They make your role essential. They make partnership the only path forward.

So use AI. Question AI. Appreciate what it can do. Recognize what it can't. And never, ever let it convince you that a pattern in data knows more about your body than you do.

Because at the end of the day, you're not trying to become an AI. You're trying to become a sovereign patient, someone who uses every tool available while staying grounded in the irreplaceable knowledge that comes from living in your own skin.

The AI Limitation Checklist

Before you bring AI-generated questions or research to your doctor, run through this checklist to ensure you're ready for partnership:

- What life context is AI missing about me?
- What recent changes in my life might affect my health?
- What matters to me that isn't in my chart?
- What subtle patterns have I noticed?
- What's my lived experience of this condition?

Technology Note

The specific AI tools mentioned in this book (ChatGPT, Claude, Gemini) are examples currently available as of the writing of this book. The principles in this chapter apply to any "Large Language Model" (LLM) AI tool, regardless of the brand name. By the time you read this, new tools may have emerged and current ones may have changed. Focus on the *type* of tool (conversational AI, symptom tracker, medical research assistant) rather than the specific company. The sovereignty principles remain constant even as the technology evolves.

7

————

ASKING BETTER QUESTIONS

If we're going to claim any real sovereignty in the exam room, we have to start with questions. Not perfect questions. Just the ones that shift you from being talked at to being included.

Sarah Discovers the Power of Preparation

Sarah sat in the waiting room of Dr. Webster's office, hands shaking slightly as she held a one-page printout. At 32, managing Type 2 diabetes for the past three years, she'd been through plenty of appointments where she nodded politely while her doctor talked, then left confused about what was supposed to happen next.

This appointment would be different. Three days ago, Sarah had dumped all her concerns into her phone's notes app. Two days ago, she'd used ChatGPT to organize that mess into a real structure: what was working, what wasn't, her three biggest questions. One day ago, she'd reviewed it, edited it, made it her own. This morning, she'd printed it out.

When Dr. Webster called her back, Sarah felt different. Instead of sitting passively, she said, "I brought a summary of what's been happening. I have three main questions. Can we make sure we cover those before we're done?"

Dr. Webster didn't sigh. She didn't glance at her watch. She read Sarah's summary, made eye contact, and leaned forward. "Good," she said. "This is really helpful. Let's work through these together."

That moment changed everything. Not because Dr. Webster had all the answers. But she welcomed Sarah's participation in the conversation.

Why Most Patients Don't Ask Questions

Before we talk about how to ask better questions, let's talk about why most of us don't.

Let's name the fear that sits in the background of so many appointments: being labeled a "problem patient." It's the fear that keeps us quiet when we're confused, or in pain, or not convinced the plan fits our life. The goal here isn't to be difficult. It's to be understood.

But there's another reason, one that's deeper than fear. From childhood, we're trained to be passive with authority figures. Doctors wear white coats. They went to medical school. They speak in terminology we don't understand. And we sit in paper gowns on exam tables, feeling small and vulnerable.

Research from the Agency for Healthcare Research and Quality (AHRQ) shows that patients who ask good questions receive better care and are more satisfied. Asking questions can help reduce medical errors, unnecessary tests, and avoidable hospital stays. But despite this evidence, most patients stay silent.

Cleveland Clinic emphasizes that patients have a right to question anyone involved with their care. Not a privilege. A right. But exercising that right requires practice, preparation, and sometimes, courage.

Before the Appointment: Preparation Is Everything

Preparation might sound like extra work. But here's the truth: organized patients get better answers. Let me walk you through the process I use now, every single time.

Three days before the appointment, I open a document and dump everything I want to discuss. Symptoms. Concerns. Medications that aren't working. Side effects I'm experiencing. Questions I've been wondering about. It's messy. It's unorganized. That's fine. The goal is just to get it out of my head and onto something I can see.

Two days before, I use AI to help me organize that mess into a one-page summary. I ask: "Help me turn these notes into a clear summary with my top three questions." The AI doesn't diagnose. It doesn't give medical advice. It just helps me communicate more clearly.

One day before, I review and edit. Sometimes AI misses important context. Sometimes it suggests questions that don't feel quite right. So I adjust. I make it mine.

The morning of the appointment, I print it out. One page. Clear sections. Top three questions highlighted. This isn't about overwhelming my doctor with information. It's about respecting his time and mine by being organized.

This preparation transforms how appointments go. Instead of trying to remember everything while sitting anxiously in the exam room, I have a roadmap. Instead of leaving and thinking, "I forgot to ask about that thing," I've already asked.

The Twelve Questions That Matter

The Agency for Healthcare Research and Quality developed a framework of essential questions through its "Questions Are the Answer" initiative. These aren't just nice-to-know information. These questions can help prevent medical errors, avoid unnecessary treatments, and help you make better decisions.

Here are the ones that have made the biggest difference in my own care.

About Your Diagnosis

"What is my diagnosis, and how do you spell it?"

This sounds obvious, but it's crucial. When I was first diagnosed with my condition, I nodded as I understood. I didn't. I went home and tried to research it, but couldn't spell it correctly, so I was reading about completely different things.

Now I ask for the spelling. I write it down. Then I ask the follow-up: "Can you explain what that means in plain language?" This isn't insulting to the doctor. It's ensuring I actually understand what we're talking about.

"What caused this?"

Understanding cause matters because it affects treatment and prevention. But sometimes the answer is: "We don't know yet." That's okay too. It's still better to know that uncertainty exists than to assume your doctor has all the answers and just isn't sharing them.

"What happens if I don't treat this?"

This is the question that changes everything. Not every condition requires immediate intervention. Understanding the natural course of a condition, what happens if you do nothing, helps you make informed decisions about whether treatment is worth its risks and costs.

About Medical Tests

"What is this test for? When will I get the results?"

Early on, I just let tests happen. Someone would say, "We're going to run some tests," and I'd say, "Okay." I didn't know what they were testing for. I didn't know when I'd find out the results. I just waited, anxious, checking my patient portal obsessively.

Now I ask: "What are we looking for? What will the results tell us? When should I expect to hear back?" This doesn't just reduce anxiety. It helps me understand what the test might reveal and what next steps might look like.

"What are the risks of this test?"

Most tests carry minimal risk. But some don't. Biopsies can cause complications. MRIs with contrast can affect kidney function. Knowing the risks helps you decide whether the test is worth doing. And sometimes when I asked about risks, my doctor would pause and say, "You know, maybe we don't need this test after all." The question itself prompted reconsideration.

About Medications

"How do you spell the name of that drug?"

Drug names are confusing. They sound similar. They're spelled in ways that don't match how they sound. When your doctor says a medication name out loud, write it down. Ask for spelling. Then when you get to the pharmacy and they hand you a bottle, you can verify it matches what was prescribed.

"What are the side effects, and which ones should prompt me to call you immediately?"

Every medication has side effects. But there's a difference between "you might feel a little nauseous" and "if you experience this symptom, go to the emergency room immediately." I learned to ask not just what side effects exist, but which ones are urgent. This helps me distinguish between expected discomfort and dangerous reactions.

"Will this medicine interact with medications I'm already taking?"

I bring a complete list of medications, including over-the-counter drugs and supplements, to every appointment. And I explicitly ask about interactions. Sometimes my doctor will say, "Let me check that," and actually look it up while I'm there. That's good doctoring.

"How long will I need to take this?"

Is this a short-term medication to address an acute problem? Or is this something you'll be taking for the rest of your life? The answer affects everything from cost to compliance to how you think about your condition.

About Treatment

"Why do I need this treatment?"

This isn't a challenge. It's a request for understanding. What is the treatment supposed to accomplish? What's the goal? How will we know if it's working? When I know the purpose, I'm more likely to follow through.

"Are there alternatives?"

Research shows that patients who understand their treatment options make better decisions. But you can't choose between options if you don't know they exist.

"What are the risks and benefits of each option?"

Every treatment is a trade-off. Benefits versus risks. Effectiveness versus side effects. Cost versus convenience. Understanding these trade-offs helps you make decisions that align with your values and your life.

The Question That Changes Everything

Those twelve questions are essential. But there's one more question that I've found more powerful than all the others combined:

"What would you do if this were you or someone you love?"

This question cuts through medical jargon and protocol. It asks your doctor to step out of their clinical role and into a human one. What would they actually choose if it were personal? That candor helps you understand not just what's medically optimal, but what's humanly reasonable.

~

Julie Learns to Frame Questions as Partnership

Julie had lived with chronic pain for five years, and in that time she'd learned something about doctors' offices. For the first five years, she attended appointments passively. Her pain management specialist would describe treatment options, and Julie would just nod and accept whatever was recommended. But the medications didn't work well, and she felt worse, not better.

Then she had a realization: she'd been so afraid of seeming difficult that she hadn't actually asked for what might help. In her next appointment with Dr. Leo Park, she tried something different. Instead of sitting passively, she said: "I know you have the expertise here, and I want to be a good partner in my care. To do that, I need to understand why we're trying this particular medication instead of the other options we discussed. Can you help me with that?"

Dr. Park didn't get defensive. He spent fifteen extra minutes walking through his reasoning. He acknowledged that the choice wasn't obvious and that different patients have different priorities. By the end, Julie understood not just what he was recommending, but why.

The difference between asking "Why are you prescribing this?" and "Can you help me understand why this medication is the best choice for my situation?" is subtle. But it transformed the conversation from confrontational to collaborative.

How to Ask Questions Without Being Labeled a "Difficult Patient"

You might be reading all these questions and thinking: "If I ask all of this, my doctor will hate me."

Here's what I've learned: It's not what you ask. It's how you ask.

Frame questions as partnership, not challenge.

Accusatory: "Why are you prescribing this?"

Collaborative: "Can you help me understand why this medication is the best choice for my situation?"

Be clear about your goal.

At the start of the appointment, say: "I have three questions I'd really like to cover today. Can we make sure we address those before we're done?" This signals that you're organized, that you're respecting their time by being focused, and that you have specific priorities.

Use the teach-back method.

At the end of the appointment, say: "Let me make sure I understood correctly. You're saying that..." Then summarize. This gives your doctor a chance to correct misunderstandings immediately, rather than you leaving with the wrong information.

All of this comes together when you walk into your doctor's office with a notebook, with organized thoughts, with clear questions, and with the confidence to say: "I need to understand this before we proceed." That's not being a difficult patient. That's being a partner.

When Your Doctor Won't Answer Questions

Let's be honest: not every doctor welcomes questions. Despite what Cleveland Clinic and AHRQ say about patient rights, some doctors still get defensive when you ask.

You might hear: "Are you questioning my expertise?" or "If you don't trust me, maybe you should find another doctor." or "Where did you read that, the internet?"

When this happens, you have a decision to make. Is this doctor willing to be a partner, or do they need you to be passive?

Sometimes it's worth one more try. You can say: "I'm not questioning your expertise. I'm trying to understand so I can be a better partner in my care. Can you help me with that?"

If they still shut you down, it might be time to find a new doctor. You have the right to question anyone involved in your care. That's not me saying it. That's Cleveland Clinic, AHRQ, and every patient advocacy organization in the country. A doctor who won't answer your questions isn't protecting their expertise. They're preventing you from being sovereign in your own health.

Mary Coordinates Care Across Multiple Providers

Mary brought two lists to her appointment—one for herself, one for her mother. Her mother sees a neurologist, a primary care physician, and a cardiologist. Until recently, none of them talked to each other.

Mary realized she had to be the coordinator. Before each of her mother's appointments, she prepared a one-page summary of what was happening: current medications, recent symptoms, concerns. She brought this to each doctor and explicitly asked them to review her mother's medications and interactions.

With Dr. Susan Chang, her mother's primary care doctor, Mary asked: "We see three different specialists. How can we make sure you all know what medications everyone is prescribing? I don't want any dangerous interactions."

Dr. Chang appreciated the question. She explained that she reviews the patient portal notes from other providers, but that it helps immensely when family members bring a summary and explicitly ask about coordination. They set up a system where Mary sends Dr. Chang an update email every month, and Dr. Chang reviews it and flags any concerns before Mary's mother's next appointment.

Mary's willingness to ask the coordination question, to be organized about it, and to engage her mother's doctors as partners transformed her mother's care. Her mother is safer, and Mary feels less overwhelmed.

How AI Helps You Ask Better Questions

AI can help you prepare for appointments in ways that weren't possible before.

1. Organize your symptoms and timeline. Instead of trying to remember when symptoms started or what makes them worse, dump everything into AI and ask it to create a timeline. "I've been tracking these symptoms. Can you help me organize them by date and severity?" This gives your doctor clear, organized information instead of scattered recollections.

2. Translate medical jargon before or after appointments. If you receive test results or a diagnosis you don't understand, you can ask AI to explain it in plain language. Then use that understanding to generate follow-up questions for your next appointment.

3. Generate questions you might not think to ask. This is where AI becomes genuinely helpful. You can describe your situation and ask: "What questions should I ask my doctor about this?" The AI will suggest questions based on best practices, questions you might not have thought of.

Then you review them, pick the ones that matter to you, add your own, and adapt them to your voice and your specific situation. The goal is AI as question assistant, not question replacement.

4. Help you understand treatment options before deciding. If your doctor presents multiple treatment options and you're overwhelmed, you can use AI to help you think through them: "I have to choose between Treatment A and Treatment B. What questions should I ask to make an informed decision?"

AI might suggest questions about long-term outcomes, side effects, cost, impact on daily life, whether the choice is reversible. These are decision-making frameworks, not medical advice.

After the Appointment: Closing the Loop

The appointment doesn't end when you leave the exam room. There's a critical step that most patients skip: follow-up.

Here's what I do: Immediately after the appointment, literally in the parking lot, I open my phone and record a voice memo. I talk through everything the doctor said while it's still fresh. Diagnosis. Treatment plan. Next steps. Questions I forgot to ask. This takes three minutes and saves hours of trying to remember later.

That evening, I review my notes and the appointment summary

from my patient portal. I use AI to help me organize this into a clear record: "Here's what happened at my appointment. Help me create a summary with action items."

If I have follow-up questions, and I usually do, I write them down. I don't call my doctor immediately. I give myself a day or two to see if the questions resolve themselves through research or reflection. If they don't, I reach out through the patient portal with specific, concise questions.

This follow-up process does two things: It ensures I actually understand what happened, and it signals to my doctor that I'm engaged and paying attention. That engagement strengthens our partnership.

From Passive Patient to Active Partner

Studies consistently show that patients who ask good questions receive better care. They have fewer medical errors. They report higher satisfaction with their treatment. And they follow through on care plans more often because they actually understand them.

But asking good questions requires practice. It requires preparation. It requires believing that you have a right to understand what's happening to your body.

You're not being difficult when you ask questions. You're being sovereign. You're exercising the right to understand. You're using AI as a preparation tool. And you're moving from passive recipient of care to active participant in it.

So start small. Pick one question from this chapter. Write it down. Bring it to your next appointment. Ask it.

See what happens when you move from passive recipient of care to active participant in it.

See what it feels like to understand what's happening to your body instead of just nodding and hoping for the best.

See what sovereignty actually looks like in practice. It looks like asking better questions. And then actually getting answers.

Create an "Appointment Preparation Form" for Your Next Visit

Print this card and bring it to your next appointment. Use it to organize your thoughts and ensure you get the information you need.

My Top 3 Questions for This Appointment

- Q1:
- Q2:
- Q3:

Symptoms or Concerns I'm Experiencing

- Current symptoms:
- Medications I'm taking:
- New side effects since last visit:

What I Need to Understand

- I really want to understand:
- What is unclear from last visit:

Next Steps (confirm before leaving)

- Treatment plan:
- When to follow up:
- Who to contact if there's a problem:

8

ORCHESTRATING YOUR
HEALTHCARE TEAM

Sarah sat in Dr. Cara Webster's office with a neat folder on her lap. Inside was her continuous glucose monitor data from the past three months, organized by her AI assistant into clear patterns. A summary from her dietitian about the nutrition changes they'd implemented together. Notes from her last cardiology appointment about her family history. And a one-page timeline showing how everything connected: better sleep had led to better glucose control, which motivated more exercise, which improved her overall metabolic health.

Dr. Webster looked up from the documents, eyebrows raised. "This is incredible," she said. "I can see exactly what's been happening between our visits. Most patients tell me they're trying to eat better and exercise more, but I don't get this kind of detail. This is the whole picture."

Sarah smiled. "I'm not doing anything special. I'm just coordinating what everyone on my team is telling me. You, my dietitian, my glucose data. AI helps me organize it all so nothing falls through the cracks."

That's the shift that happens when you move from passive patient to active conductor: You realize nobody else is connecting the dots. Your primary care physician sees you once a quarter. Your specialist sees you every few months. Your pharmacist reviews prescriptions as they come in. Each one is excellent at their role. But who's making sure they're all working together?

You are. And increasingly, AI can help you be a partner to do that work without it becoming a second job.

THE HIDDEN GAP IN HEALTHCARE COORDINATION

Nobody tells you this when you're managing a chronic condition, navigating multiple specialists, or just trying to optimize your health: Nobody is coordinating your care except you.

Your specialist is focused on their area of expertise. Your primary care physician is managing your overall health and preventive care. Your pharmacist is reviewing prescriptions as they come in. Each one is excellent at what they do. But who's making sure they're all working together? Who's ensuring the medication your specialist prescribed doesn't interact with what your primary care physician recommended? Who's noticing when one provider's advice contradicts another's?

You are.

Care coordination failures contribute to thousands of preventable deaths and hospitalizations annually in the United States. The problem isn't incompetent providers. It's fragmented systems where specialists work in silos and nobody has the complete picture.

Except you. You have the complete picture because you are the complete picture.

And increasingly, AI can help you organize that picture in ways that make coordination possible. Not as a burden, but as a natural part of managing your health.

JULIE'S WAKE-UP CALL

Julie, you know her well by now as she manages chronic pain. She sees Dr. Leo Park (her pain management specialist), Dr. Susan Chang (her primary care physician), and sometimes Dr. Noor Ahmed when her symptoms flare. Three different doctors, three separate medical records systems, three sets of prescriptions filled at different pharmacies based on which one seemed cheapest that month.

Julie thought she was being responsible. She followed each doctor's instructions. She took her medications as prescribed. What she didn't realize was that nobody had the complete picture. Not even her.

Dr. Leo Park prescribed a new pain medication to improve her function. Dr. Susan Chang, unaware of the change, adjusted Julie's blood pressure medication during a routine visit. Dr. Noor Ahmed added an anti-inflammatory during a flare-up. Each prescription made sense in isolation. Together, they caused Julie to feel light-headed, confused, and exhausted for weeks.

She blamed herself. She thought she wasn't handling the pain well enough. She wondered if her condition was getting worse. She almost cancelled plans with her two kids because she felt too foggy to drive safely. Then her mother visited and pointed out what Julie had missed: she'd gotten noticeably less like herself since starting the new medication.

At her next appointment with Dr. Chang, Julie pulled out her phone and showed her all three medication lists. "Will these interact?" she asked. Dr. Chang's expression changed immediately. "Yes," she said quietly. "Let's call Dr. Park and coordinate this. This is exactly the kind of thing that slips through the cracks."

Julie left the hospital with an important lesson learned and a new system. She started using a medication tracking app to maintain a master medication list. Everything she takes, when she takes it, what it's for, which doctor prescribed it. Every medication change gets logged immediately. Before any appointment, her app generates a current medication summary that includes everything: prescriptions, over-the-counter medications, and supplements.

Now, when any provider wants to prescribe something new, Julie pulls out her phone and shows them the complete list. "Will this interact with anything I'm currently taking?" she asks. And crucially, she uses a single pharmacy for everything, so her pharmacist Raj can also review the complete picture.

Many medication errors occur when different providers work with partial information about your medications. Different providers working with incomplete information about what patients are actually taking, especially when this takes place over multiple health systems. Julie's story isn't unusual. It's frighteningly common.

The difference now is that AI makes comprehensive medication tracking effortless. Julie doesn't maintain spreadsheets or complex systems. She just tells her AI assistant when something changes, and it keeps the master list current. Simple. Automatic. Potentially lifesaving.

BUILDING YOUR CORE TEAM

When you think about your healthcare team, it's much bigger than just the doctors you see. Each member has a specific role, and together they create something stronger than any individual provider could offer alone.

YOUR PRIMARY CARE PHYSICIAN: THE FOUNDATION

Your primary care physician is the most important member of your healthcare team. Here's why: They see the whole picture. Not just one organ system or condition, but your overall health across time. Annual physicals, preventive screenings, vaccinations, and those random concerns that don't quite fit into a specialty ("Is this mole normal?" "Should I be worried about this knee pain?").

But here's what makes a good PCP truly invaluable: They serve as the bridge between specialists. When your cardiologist makes one recommendation and your endocrinologist makes another, your PCP can help determine whether those recommendations are compatible and safe. They're the one provider who should know about everything - every specialist you see, every medication you take, every health concern you're managing.

Think of your PCP as the conductor of your healthcare orchestra. The specialists are virtuosos on their particular instruments, but your PCP ensures they're all playing the same symphony.

The challenge? Your PCP only sees you once or twice a year, typically for 15-20 minutes. They're managing hundreds of patients, each with their own complex health situations. They can't possibly remember the nuances of your case between visits unless you help them.

This is where your role as coordinator becomes crucial. When you walk into your PCP's office with an organized summary of what's happened since your last visit - what specialists you've seen, what medications have changed, what symptoms you're tracking - you transform that 15-minute appointment into a productive partnership. You're not asking your PCP to remember everything. You're bringing them the information they need to help you effectively.

A strong relationship with your PCP is worth investing in. They're your advocate, your coordinator, and often the first person who can spot connections between seemingly unrelated health issues. Don't underestimate how valuable this relationship is to your long-term health.

YOUR SPECIALIST (IF YOU HAVE ONE): THE EXPERT

If you're managing a specific condition, you might work with a specialist who understands the nuances of that particular area. Cardiology, endocrinology, neurology, oncology. They know the latest research, the treatment options, the warning signs to watch for.

But specialists typically see you every three to six months for 15-20 minutes. They can't possibly know everything that happens between visits unless you tell them effectively.

YOUR PHARMACIST: THE MEDICATION SAFETY EXPERT

After Julie's experience, she learned something crucial: Pharmacists aren't just pill dispensers. They're medication experts who often catch dangerous interactions that busy doctors might miss.

Many pharmacies offer comprehensive medication reviews. A service where your pharmacist sits down with you to review everything you're taking. Not just prescriptions, but also supplements, over-the-counter medications, even herbal teas or vitamins.

Julie brings her AI-generated medication list to these reviews. Everything she's taking, when she takes it, what it's for, which provider prescribed it, when it was started. Her pharmacist Raj can quickly scan the complete picture and identify potential problems.

Last year, Raj caught a potential interaction between Julie's prescription medication and a magnesium supplement she'd started taking for sleep. Dr. Park hadn't asked about supplements. Dr. Chang didn't know she'd started it. But Raj saw the complete picture and flagged the risk before it became a problem.

Pharmacist-led medication reviews prevent thousands of adverse drug events annually. Ask your pharmacy about scheduling a medication review. Many offer this service for free, and it's one of the most valuable safety nets you can add to your team.

YOUR TRUSTED ADVISOR: THE OBSERVER

Whether it's a family member, close friend, or partner, having someone who knows you well can be invaluable. They're not health-care professionals, but they're people who see you regularly and can notice subtle changes you might miss from the inside.

The truth about living with a health condition is this: You can't always see yourself clearly. When changes happen gradually - your energy declining week by week, your mood shifting, your thinking getting a bit foggier - you adapt without realizing it. You tell yourself you're just tired, or stressed, or getting older. You normalize what's actually a warning sign.

But the people close to you? They notice.

They notice you're not laughing as much. They notice you're forgetting things you used to remember easily. They notice you're moving more carefully, or sleeping more, or seeming distant. They notice you've stopped doing activities you used to love. These subtle shifts often appear long before lab results change or symptoms become obvious enough to report to a doctor.

Julie's mother had noticed she'd become "noticeably less like herself" after starting new medications. Julie had blamed herself, thinking she wasn't handling her pain well. But her mother saw the medication interaction from the outside in a way Julie couldn't see from the inside.

What Trusted Advisors Can Do:

Notice patterns you can't see. When you live with chronic symptoms every day, it's hard to know if you're getting worse, staying the same, or actually improving. Someone who sees you regularly but doesn't live in your body can provide that perspective.

Advocate when you can't. When you're exhausted, in pain, or overwhelmed, having someone who can speak up for you in medical settings is powerful. They can ask the questions you forget. They can push back when you're too tired to advocate for yourself.

Provide accountability and support. Managing chronic conditions requires consistent effort - taking medications, tracking symptoms, following treatment plans. Having someone who checks in, who reminds you, who encourages you when you're frustrated, makes that burden lighter.

Attend appointments with you. Two sets of ears hear more than one. When you're anxious or overwhelmed in a medical appointment, you might miss important information. Your trusted advisor can take notes, ask clarifying questions, and help you remember what was discussed.

How AI Helps Trusted Advisors Contribute:

Your trusted advisor doesn't need medical expertise to be helpful. AI can give them simple ways to contribute:

- They can help you record voice memos after appointments if you're too tired
- They can add their observations to your health log: "Noticed Dan seemed more confused than usual this week"
- They can review your AI-generated appointment summaries to make sure nothing important was missed
- They can help you prepare questions before appointments
- They can track patterns you might not notice yourself

Important: Your trusted advisor should support your autonomy, not take over your healthcare decisions. The best advisors observe, advocate, and assist - but they respect that this is your health, your body, your decisions.

Not everyone has a trusted advisor, and that's okay. But if you do have someone willing to be observant and supportive, don't hesitate to bring them into your healthcare team. Give them permission to speak up when they notice changes. Ask them to come to important appointments. Let them help you stay organized when you're overwhelmed.

The healthcare system often treats patients as isolated individuals. But health happens in the context of relationships. The people who know you best are part of your care team, whether the medical system recognizes it or not.

Your Support Group (If You Have One): The Experience Experts

If you're managing a specific condition, connecting with others who share that experience can provide insights that even the best doctors can't offer. Support groups, whether in-person or online, give you access to practical wisdom from people living with what you're going through.

Many people with chronic conditions find that fellow patients' insights are as valuable as professional medical advice for managing day-to-day challenges. Not for diagnosis or treatment decisions, but for the practical navigation of living with a condition.

Mary's Team Transformation

Mary describes herself as "not tech-savvy." She works full-time as a marketing manager while managing her own health through Dr. Aisha Chen (primary care), a specialist who manages her chronic condition, and a physical therapist.

"I couldn't keep track of who told me what," she said. "Dr. Chang would adjust my medication, but I'd forget to mention it to my physical therapist, and then I couldn't figure out why my treatment wasn't working as well as it should."

Her daughter suggested trying a simple AI system. Just use voice memos on her phone to track what each provider told her.

Mary was skeptical. "I barely know how to text," she said. "How am I supposed to use artificial intelligence?"

But her daughter showed her it was simpler than she thought. After each medical appointment, Mary would record a voice memo in her car before driving home: "Dr. Chang said my blood pressure is better. She's happy with my current medication. She wants to see me in six months. Also mentioned my vitamin D is still a bit low, even with supplements."

That's it. No typing, no complex app, no medical terminology. Just talking to her phone like she was telling someone what happened.

Her AI assistant transcribed these memos and organized them by provider and date. When Mary had an upcoming appointment, her daughter would help her ask the AI: "What did Dr. Chang tell me at my last visit? What questions did I want to ask her?"

The AI would pull up the relevant information. Mary started bringing these AI-generated summaries to her appointments printed on paper. One page that said what happened last time and what questions she had for this visit.

Her providers noticed the change immediately. "Mary, this is so helpful," Dr. Webster said. "I can see exactly what Dr. Chang discussed and how you've been responding. This helps me coordinate my recommendations with hers."

Over six months, Mary's health coordination transformed. She stopped missing appointments because her AI assistant sent her reminders. She stopped getting confused about medications because she had a clear, current list. She stopped feeling overwhelmed because information was organized and accessible.

"I'm not tech-savvy," Mary insists. "But I can talk to my phone. And having someone, even if it's an AI someone, keeping track of everything has changed my life. I feel like I'm in control again."

The United States ranks last among high-income countries in care coordination. This isn't because American patients are less capable. It's because our fragmented system makes coordination extraordinarily difficult. Simple AI tools can bridge that gap for anyone willing to speak into their phone after medical appointments.

AI as Organizational Tool, Not Replacement for Thinking

I want to be specific about what AI does and doesn't do in healthcare coordination:

1. AI does not diagnose conditions
2. AI does not recommend treatments

3. AI does not replace medical judgment
4. AI does not make healthcare decisions

What AI does, brilliantly, is organize information so you can coordinate your care more effectively.

THINK of it like having a highly competent personal assistant who:

1. Maintains your complete medication list
2. Organizes your symptom logs into readable timelines
3. Tracks which provider said what and when
4. Generates summaries before appointments
5. Helps you remember questions you wanted to ask
6. Keeps all your health information accessible and organized

You still make all the decisions. You still have the conversations with your providers. You still determine what information is relevant and what actions to take. But instead of trying to remember everything or maintain complex organizational systems, you have AI handling the clerical coordination work.

Starting Your Team Audit: A Practical Framework

If you're feeling overwhelmed by the idea of coordinating your healthcare team, start with a simple audit. You don't need fancy systems or complex tools. You just need to understand your current situation.

Who's on Your Team Now?

Write down every healthcare provider you currently see:

1. Primary care physician
2. Specialists (all of them, even if you only see them occasionally)
3. Pharmacist
4. Any allied health professionals (physical therapist, dietitian, mental health provider)
5. Trusted family members or friends who observe your health

For each provider, note:

1. When you last saw them
2. When your next appointment is scheduled
3. What they're helping you manage
4. How you currently communicate with them

This simple exercise often reveals gaps. Maybe you haven't seen your PCP in over a year. Maybe you have three specialists but they never communicate with each other.

Simple AI-Assisted Tracking Template

You don't need complex systems. You need consistent, simple practices:

1. Create a central health log. A single document or note where all health information lives.
2. After every medical appointment, spend two minutes creating a voice memo: "Just saw [provider name]. They said [key findings]. They recommended [treatment or changes]. They want [follow-up actions]. Next appointment [date]."
3. Let your AI assistant transcribe and organize these memos chronologically.
4. Maintain a current medication list. Every time you start, stop, or change a medication or supplement, tell your AI: "Started/stopped/changed [medication name, dosage, frequency, reason]."
5. Before any appointment, ask your AI to summarize relevant information since your last visit with that specific provider.
6. Monthly review: Ask your AI, "What health events or changes have happened this month? Do any team

members need to be updated about changes other
providers made?"

That's it. Voice memos after appointments using a tool like Audio-Pen, Drafts or if you have a Mac tools like Voice Memos. Medication updates as they happen. Pre-appointment summaries. Monthly coordination check-ins. No complex apps. No medical expertise required. No hours of work.

The Power of Being the Conductor

When you accept that you need to be the conductor of your healthcare team, not because you want to, but because the fragmented system requires it, something shifts. You stop feeling overwhelmed by healthcare chaos and start feeling like an active participant in your own care.

You're not a medical expert. You don't diagnose your conditions or prescribe your treatments. But you are the world's foremost expert on your own body, your own experience, your own health journey.

You're the person who knows what all your providers have said. You're the person who experiences how different treatments interact. You're the person who can spot patterns across time. You're the person who can ensure information flows between disconnected systems.

With AI assistance, you can fulfill that role without it becoming a second job. You can coordinate care effectively while still living your life. You can ensure your healthcare team works together instead of in silos.

This isn't how healthcare should work. Ideally, systems would be integrated, information would flow seamlessly, and patients wouldn't need to coordinate their own care. But until that future arrives, you have AI tools that make patient-led coordination possible.

Being the conductor of your healthcare team isn't an extra burden. It's a form of self-protection. And with AI assistance, it's a role anyone can fill, regardless of technical skill, medical knowledge, or organizational ability.

You just need to start. Pick one simple practice. Maybe maintaining a complete medication list, or recording brief voice memos after appointments. Start small. Build gradually. Let AI handle the organization while you handle the coordination.

Your healthcare team is more effective when someone connects the dots. That someone is you. And now, you have tools that make that coordination sustainable.

Your Care Team Roster

Create your own care team roster to keep track of everyone involved in your care. Keep it updated and bring it to every appointment so each provider knows who else is on your team.

Your roster should include:

1. Primary Care Provider (name, practice, phone, patient portal, role in your care)
2. Specialists (name, specialty, phone, role in your care)
3. Pharmacy (name, phone, pharmacist you talk to)
4. Other Team Members (physical therapist, mental health provider, etc.)

When a provider asks "Who else are you seeing?" use this roster to ensure they know about your full team. When you get new test results or a diagnosis, note which other providers should be informed. When medications change, mark which team members need to know.

This simple roster makes you the conductor. Keep it updated. Share it generously. It's how disconnected specialists become a coordinated team.

9

—————

YOUR DATA, YOUR RULES

Who owns the data your body creates? Most of us assume the answer is simple until we realize how much of that data is being generated outside the clinic and outside our awareness. Some of it is helpful. Some of it is sensitive. And some of it starts moving the moment it's created.

Sarah is sitting at her kitchen table at 6 AM, coffee in hand, watching the data accumulate on her phone. Her smartwatch has been tracking her sleep all night, and this morning the numbers are rough: four hours total, disrupted sleep, lots of time awake in the middle of the night.

It was 2 a.m. again. Sarah's blood sugar had woken her—the nights like this, where her blood sugar swings make sleep nearly impossible, are familiar. She has apps tracking her glucose patterns, her sleep quality, her activity levels. She has a continuous glucose monitor on her arm sending readings to her phone every five minutes. She has a fitness tracker logging her heart rate, her steps, her stress levels throughout the day.

What she does not have is any real sense of what happens to all this data once it leaves her devices. Where does it go? Who sees it? Can it be used against her?

Sarah has never thought much about it. The apps promised to help her manage her health better. The devices were designed to give her visibility into her own body. The companies behind them seemed legitimate. So she used them, trusted them, and assumed the data was as protected as her medical records in her doctor's office.

But this morning, reading an article on her phone while waiting for her coffee to cool, she learned something that made her set the cup down untouched: The moment your health data leaves your body and enters a device or app, it stops being just yours. It becomes a commodity. It can be analyzed, sold, shared, and used in ways you never imagined or consented to.

The article mentioned numbers. Incomprehensible numbers. A complete health data profile can be worth between $500 and $1,000 on the open market. For someone like Sarah, with years of detailed diabetes management data, that value increases dramatically. Her data is worth thousands to insurance companies, pharmaceutical firms, and marketers who want to understand people living with chronic conditions.

Sarah set her phone down and looked at her glucose monitor. The device on her arm, which she trusted to help her stay healthy, was collecting information worth money to someone else. And she was not seeing a penny of it.

Sarah didn't know it, but every time she logged her blood sugar in that free app, she was feeding a profile. That profile would be packaged, sold, and analyzed by companies she'd never heard of. It would help calculate whether she was "too risky" for affordable insurance, a good candidate for pharmaceutical marketing, or just another data point in an actuarial model predicting her future costs. Her vulnerability had literal monetary value to entities who would use that information in ways she'd never see or consent to. This is what makes the extraction paradigm so troubling: it takes advantage of our desire to take care of ourselves.

What Really Happens to Your Health Data

Here is what most of us do not realize when we hand over health data to apps and devices: Oversight is fragmented. Protection is incomplete. The legal framework has significant gaps that the average person rarely thinks about.

HIPAA (the Health Insurance Portability and Accountability Act) is often treated like a comprehensive privacy shield. It sounds protective. It feels protective. But in reality, HIPAA only covers covered entities, which means hospitals, doctors, insurance companies, and pharmacies. The moment your health data enters a device or app that is not directly part of your medical care, HIPAA protections largely disappear.

That fitness tracker? Not covered by HIPAA. That glucose monitoring app? Not covered. That meditation app tracking your stress and mood? Not covered. The AI assistant you are using to organize your symptoms? Not covered.

This creates what researchers call the HIPAA gap, an enormous blind spot where the most valuable, most granular health data exists with minimal legal privacy protection. A person with a chronic condition generates approximately 1.2 million data points per year from wearables, apps, and connected health devices. Almost none of that falls under HIPAA protection.

And that data is worth real money to real companies. The global health data market was valued at $34.7 billion in 2023 and is projected to reach $127.3 billion by 2030. That is not healthcare spending or research funding. That is the market for buying and selling health-related data. Your data. My data. Data about people just trying to manage their health.

Who buys this data? Pharmaceutical companies trying to identify drug candidates and target marketing. Insurance companies refining risk models and identifying high-cost patients. Employers assessing workforce health trends. Marketers targeting health-conscious consumers. Data brokers creating detailed health profiles to sell to the highest bidder.

What does that look like in practice? Let us look at a woman named Julie.

When Data Becomes Discrimination

Julie had been living with chronic pain for five years. Some days are manageable. Some days the pain makes everything harder. She uses technology extensively to manage her condition: a fitness tracker to monitor her activity levels without overdoing it, apps to track her pain patterns, a smartwatch to see how activity affects her sleep.

A year ago, Julie applied for a promotion at her company. She was the obvious choice: solid performance history, strong relationships with her team, ready for more responsibility. The promotion included enrollment in the company's executive health program.

The program was framed as a premium benefit, a perk that came with leadership roles. Comprehensive health screenings, wellness coaching, and the required use of a specific fitness tracker that fed data back to the company's wellness dashboard. HR made it clear: it is part of the benefits package. All executives participate.

Julie was hesitant. She was already using her own tracker, carefully configured to keep her data private. But she wanted the promotion. She had earned it. She agreed to the program.

Three weeks into her new role, her boss called her into his office. His tone was carefully sympathetic as he turned his laptop toward her. He showed her sleep data displayed in charts and graphs. Days with disrupted sleep. Nights with multiple awakenings. Long stretches to fall asleep. Activity patterns that did not match what HR considered optimal.

'We are concerned about your ability to handle the stress of this executive role,' he continued, his voice taking on that rehearsed tone of concern. 'Leadership positions require peak performance, and your wellness metrics suggest you might not be getting the recovery you need.'

Julie felt her face flush. Her sleep patterns, driven by her chronic pain condition, were being presented as evidence that she was not capable of doing her job. 'This is a medical issue,' she said carefully. 'It is part of my chronic pain condition. You cannot use health data to make employment decisions.'

'This is not health data,' her boss replied. 'It is wellness data. You consented to share it when you joined the program. We are not making employment decisions based on medical conditions. We are simply concerned about your wellness metrics.'

Julie was mortified and quickly consulted with an employment lawyer who was a friend of a friend. The answer was frustrating: the wellness program existed in a legal gray zone. The data came from a voluntary wellness device rather than medical records, so it was not clearly protected under the Americans with Disabilities Act. Because she had consented to share the data, the company argued they had permission to use it for wellness support.

She kept the promotion, but only after removing herself from the wellness program and filing a formal complaint with HR. The experience left her shaken. She had thought tracking her data was empowering. Instead, she had handed her employer a window into her body's most intimate struggles. Struggles that had nothing to do with her professional capabilities but could be weaponized against her nonetheless.

The Insurance Trap: Mary's Experience

Mary is 58 years old, a working professional who is also the primary caregiver for her mother, who was diagnosed with Alzheimer's five years ago. The stress is relentless. Mary uses a fitness tracker to monitor her own health, to catch signs of stress, to prove to herself that she is taking care of her own wellbeing while caring for someone else.

When Mary applied for life insurance, the agent asked about fitness tracking. Mary was proud to say yes. Her data would show good health habits. The agent smiled. 'Great. We partner with wearable companies. If you consent to share your data, we can offer you lower premiums based on verified healthy behaviors.'

The discount looked good. Mary consented without reading the fine print.

Two months later, Mary had a month of chaos. Her mother had a health scare. Mary reduced her exercise routine, slept poorly, had nights when stress kept her awake. She was still active, still healthy, but her tracker showed decreased activity and poor sleep patterns.

The insurance company noticed. They reduced her premium discount, claiming decreased activity levels and suboptimal sleep patterns had changed her risk profile. Mary tried to explain that this was a temporary stress response to her mother's health crisis, that she was fine, that her underlying health was still good.

The company's response was clinical. 'Your average daily step count decreased by 18%. Your sleep efficiency score dropped below our healthy threshold for multiple weeks. These changes affect your risk profile. The algorithm adjusts premiums accordingly. You can improve your discount by increasing your activity levels.'

Mary tried to opt out of data sharing. The insurance company's response: 'You can discontinue data sharing. Your premium will revert to the standard rate, which is 15% higher than your current reduced rate.'

Mary found herself in an impossible choice. Stop sharing data and pay significantly more for insurance. Keep sharing data and live under constant algorithmic judgment. Her baseline premium had been secretly inflated to create a discount that required perpetual surveillance to maintain.

What started as helpful health tracking had transformed into a system where every moment of rest, every busy season at work, every night of stress was monetized and measured against an algorithm.

Empowerment: What Data Sovereignty Actually Means

After learning about what happens to health data in systems like these, you might feel like you have no options. Use the apps and risk surveillance. Do not use them and miss out on health management tools. There is no good choice.

But there are actually concrete steps you can take right now to reclaim control over your health data. Data sovereignty does not mean abandoning all technology. It means making informed choices about what you use, what you share, and what you demand from companies that want access to your information.

Know What Data You Are Creating

Start with an inventory. Write down every app, every device, every platform that touches your health data. For each one, ask: What data does this collect? Where does that data go? Who has access to it? What are they allowed to do with it? Can I delete it?

You can use an AI assistant to help. Upload the privacy policy and ask specific questions: Does this company sell my data to third parties? Can they share my data with insurance companies? What happens to my data if I delete my account?

The results might surprise you. Most health apps reserve the right to share or sell data to third parties. Many retain data indefinitely even after you delete your account. Some share data with partners whose identities they do not even disclose.

Choose Tools That Respect Your Sovereignty

Once you understand what data you are creating and where it is going, you can start making different choices. There are smaller companies, privacy-focused tools, and alternatives to the big mainstream platforms. They often cost more. They sometimes have fewer features. But they keep your data yours.

Look for specific features: local data storage, end-to-end encryption, clear data deletion policies, and explicit commitments never to sell user data. If a health technology product is free or suspiciously cheap, ask yourself how they are making money. Often the answer is by selling your data.

You might use a fitness device that stores all data locally instead of sending it to company servers. You might use a symptom-tracking app that encrypts everything on your device. You might choose an AI assistant service that does not store conversations after the session ends.

These choices require more research and sometimes cost more money. But they give you actual control over data that represents your body and your health.

Demand Granular Control

Real data sovereignty means granular control. Share your step count but not your sleep data. Allow one app to access your heart rate for workout optimization, but not to share it with third parties. Permit research use of your anonymized data but prohibit commercial use.

Some platforms offer this. Most do not. When you encounter an accept all or decline all data sharing agreement, choose decline. See what actually happens. Often the required data sharing is not required at all. It is just profitable for the company.

This process takes effort. Auditing your data settings quarterly, reviewing privacy policy updates, revoking unnecessary permissions. But it is the price of data sovereignty in a system designed to separate you from control of your own information.

Partnership: Working with Your Healthcare Team

Here is the thing: many healthcare providers do not understand that patients often have far more accurate data about their conditions than what is in medical records. Sarah's glucose patterns from her continuous monitor. Julie's detailed pain and sleep tracking. Mary's stress response patterns from her wearable.

When you work with clinicians, you can bring this data to the conversation. Dr. Cara Webster, an endocrinologist Sarah works with, has learned to ask specifically what data her patients are tracking. 'I can see your glucose readings from when you come in,' Dr. Webster tells Sarah. 'But you are tracking patterns I never see. Bring that to our visits. That information helps me understand your condition in ways the medical record does not.'

This works best when there is clarity about what data you are willing to share and what you are not. You might ask Dr. Leo Park, Julie's pain specialist, to help interpret patterns from your activity tracker without that data automatically going into your medical record, where it might be sold, shared, or used against you.

And you can ask your clinician to be thoughtful about what gets documented in the medical record itself. Mary asked her primary care doctor, Dr. Susan Chang, whether the note about her stress and sleep disruption during her mother's health crisis was essential to her ongoing care. 'It matters for context,' Dr. Susan Chang said. 'But we can note that you are managing stress through your care routine without a detailed description of the specific stressors.'

The goal is partnership without oversharing. Your clinicians have a responsibility to help you manage your health. You have the right to determine what data supports that work and what data goes beyond your care into systems that might misuse it.

When you bring this up with your healthcare team, use language like: 'I have been tracking this specific data that I think would be helpful for you to understand. What is the best way to share this without it going into permanent records that insurance might see?' Most clinicians will respect this boundary.

Some healthcare systems are starting to get it right. Increasingly, hospitals and clinics are implementing granular data controls where you can choose which providers see which portions of your records, permit research use for specific disease categories while prohibiting others, and default to maximum privacy with explicit opt-in for data sharing beyond direct care.

Your Data. Your Rules.

If you are feeling overwhelmed by all of this, I understand. The data landscape is intentionally complex, designed to exhaust you into clicking accept without reading or thinking.

But you can start small. Pick one health app or device you use regularly. Upload its privacy policy to an AI assistant and ask what the company does with your data. Read the answer. Decide if you are comfortable with it.

Before you agree to share health data with your employer's wellness program or your insurance company's discount program, ask yourself: What am I actually consenting to? What happens to this data? Who sees it? Can it be used against me?

Your health data represents your body. It tells your story. It has commercial value to others, but it has personal value to you that cannot be measured in dollars.

You have the right to control it. You have the right to know where it goes. You have the right to demand better than accept all or decline all.

That right, that sovereignty, starts with a simple refusal. The next time you are asked to hand over your health data, pause. Read what you are agreeing to. Ask yourself if it is worth it.

And if it is not, have the courage to click decline.

YOUR DATA. YOUR RULES. NEXT STEPS.

Create a form like this in Google Docs for your next health visit. I call it my "Data Privacy Conversation."

Questions to Ask

- *List the health data you currently track (apps, devices, wearables):*
- Example: sleep, heart rate, steps, seizures, pain levels, mood, medication timing, blood pressure, glucose
- *Ask your clinician:*
- "I track [specific data]. Would any of this be helpful in understanding my symptoms or treatment response?"
- *Decide what you're comfortable sharing:*
- Data I'm comfortable having documented in my medical record:
- Data I'm comfortable discussing verbally, but prefer not to have documented in detail:
- *If you want to limit documentation, ask directly:*
- "Can we discuss this data without documenting the specific details in my permanent record?"
- "If it needs to be documented, can we keep it high-level?"
- *After the visit, review your visit note and portal record:*
- Look for mentions of your tracking data.
- If something feels inaccurate or too detailed, consider requesting a correction or clarification.
- *One important nuance:* Clinicians may not be able to honor every request to keep something out of the record, especially if it affects safety, medical decision-making, or legal documentation.

10

DEFINING WHAT MATTERS TO YOU

This chapter is going to be different. There are no tools here, no scripts for doctor conversations, no AI shortcuts to make the work easier. This is the chapter where we go inward. This is the very soul of patient sovereignty.

Because here's the truth: No one can tell you what should matter most in your healthcare journey. Not your doctor, no matter how skilled. Not your family, no matter how much they love you. Not this book, no matter how many frameworks it offers. This is work only you can do—the deeply personal, sometimes uncomfortable process of defining what you actually want from your life with this condition.

You can involve the people closest to you. You should listen to medical expertise. But ultimately, you're the one who has to live in your body, experience the side effects, make the daily accommodations, and wake up each morning with the consequences of your healthcare decisions. This is your life. These are your priorities to define.

If that feels heavy, it should. This is the hardest work in the book. It requires honesty that might be painful. It asks you to confront tradeoffs you'd rather not think about. It demands clarity about what you're willing to sacrifice and what you're not.

But it's also the most important work you'll do. Because until you know what matters to you—really know it, not what should matter or what matters to others—you can't effectively advocate for yourself. You can't evaluate treatment options. You can't have the conversations that will transform your healthcare from something that happens to you into something you actively shape.

So take your time with this chapter. Sit with the questions. Let yourself feel whatever comes up. This isn't about finding the "right" answers. It's about finding your answers.

When you're living with a complex medical condition, there's a question you should be asking yourself that no one else may ask you. Not because they don't care, but because there are no easy answers. Or in the case of your healthcare providers they simply don't have time. Your doctors are managing dozens of patients, rushing through appointments, focused on short-term clinical outcomes and medication adjustments. They're asking about symptoms, side effects, lab results. All important things. But few people ask the most important question: What are your goals for your life with this condition? If nothing else very few people remind you that these are important questions you need to be asking yourself.

I remember the moment I realized I'd been managing my health for years without ever answering this question. I'd been so focused on just surviving; managing the symptoms, adjusting to medications, trying to function through the fog, that I hadn't thought about what I actually wanted my life to look like. What was I trying to achieve beyond 'not getting worse' and 'avoiding the worst outcomes'? What was even possible, and how would I get there?

If someone had asked me what my goal was, I would have said, 'I want to get better.' The words would have felt automatic, reflexive, just like the expected answer.

But 'getting better' isn't a goal. It's a wish. A vague hope. And vague hopes don't drive treatment decisions. They don't help you evaluate whether a medication's side effects are worth its benefits. They don't guide you when you're choosing between multiple treatment options with different tradeoffs. They don't empower you to be sovereign over your own healthcare.

It took me too long to realize this. I kept waiting for my healthcare team to tell me what I should be aiming for, what success should look like, what 'better' meant. But they couldn't tell me that. They could tell me what the medications might do, what the clinical outcomes looked like, and what the research showed. But only I could define what I actually wanted my life to look like.

Real sovereignty requires something more specific: You need to know what matters to you. Not what should matter, not what matters to other patients or to your doctor or to some generic 'reasonable person.' What matters to you, specifically, given your life, your values, your circumstances, your priorities.

This chapter is about that process—the deeply personal, sometimes uncomfortable work of defining what you actually want from your healthcare journey. Because until you know what matters to you, you can't effectively advocate for it. And if you can't advocate for what matters, you're not sovereign. You're just along for the ride.

This isn't work your doctor will do for you. They're focused on managing your condition. You need to focus on managing your life. And that starts with asking yourself a question that has no medical answer: What do I actually want from my healthcare?

The Tyranny of 'Getting Better'

When you're sick or injured, everyone asks the same question: 'Are you getting better?'

It's well-meaning. It's natural. And it's completely useless as a framework for making healthcare decisions.

'Getting better' is too broad, too undefined, too open to interpretation. Better than what, before I got sick? Better in which way? Better according to whose definition, my immediate family, my extended family, my employer, who?

After my brain injury, different people had wildly different ideas of what 'getting better' meant for me:

One neurologist measured it by seizure frequency. If I went from two seizures per week to one, I was getting better. The side effects, the exhaustion, the cognitive fog, the tremor in my hands, were acceptable tradeoffs for reduced seizure activity. Sadly, no one told me this.

For some it may be defined by your employer as being able to return to work. Could you sit at a computer for eight hours? Could you participate in meetings? If yes, you were better enough. The fact that you came home so depleted you could barely function in the evenings didn't factor into their calculus.

Your family may measure it by whether you seem more like your pre-injury self. Was your personality and sense of humor returning? Could you engage in conversations the way you used to? The medical details mattered less to them than whether they were getting 'the old you' back.

All of these are valid perspectives. None of them are wrong. But they are all different, and they sometimes can feel in conflict. A medication that reduces seizures might increase cognitive fog. A work schedule that satisfies your employer might leave you unable to engage with family. 'Getting better' means different things to different people and you are caught in the middle, trying to satisfy everyone while having no clear sense of what you are actually trying to achieve for yourself.

The televisit is vivid. My neurologist had left for the day, and we were speaking while he was at home with his family. Here I was sitting in the lobby of my primary medical center seeing another provider while my specialist was at home. We had reached a point that a major decision had to be made. My seizure events had generally stabilized, but they hadn't left. The realization came as my neurologist shared my seizures would probably never stop. I had reached normal as normal could be, for me. He said we could possibly switch me to a newer medication, but there was no telling it would help and potentially it could create more side effects with greater possible risks for long-term risk of dementia. No amount of effort or research would help answer this question. I had a choice to make.

'What do you think?' he asked.

I had no idea what I thought. The sadness rising in my chest. Both options sounded terrible in different ways. The risk of potentially more seizures versus more brain fog and memory loss. Which mattered more? I didn't know. I'd been so busy trying to be a 'good patient'—knowledgeable, respectful, willing to consider whatever the doctor recommended—that I'd never stopped to consider what I actually wanted my life to look like. I had reached the end of the road. What did I want?

The neurologist waited, watching me struggle. Finally, he said something that changed everything:

'You're the one who has to live with whichever decision we make. Not me. Not your family. You. So what do you need your brain to do? What's most important to you in your daily life?'

It was the first time a doctor had asked me to define my own priorities rather than simply optimizing for a clinical outcome. And I had no answer ready. I'd spent years learning about my condition, studying my symptoms and lab results, learning about seizure medications, about treatment protocols, but I'd spent zero time thinking about what I actually valued, what I was willing to sacrifice and what I wasn't.

That night, I started making a list.

What I Actually Needed My Brain to Do

Sitting with a cup of coffee, glancing out the window with a notebook, I wrote the question at the top of the page:

What do I need my brain to do?

The first answers came quickly, almost reflexively: Think clearly. Remember things. Not have seizures. Standard stuff. But as I sat with the question longer, more specific needs emerged:

I needed to be able to write—not just type words, but think through complex ideas and articulate them coherently. Writing had always been how I processed the world, how I made sense of chaos. A

medication that dulled my ability to find the right words or follow a
train of thought would fundamentally change who I was.

I needed to be able to have real conversations with my family. Not
just be physically present, but mentally engaged. Able to follow what
my partner was saying, remember the context from previous conversations, contribute meaningfully. Connection mattered more to me
than productivity.

I needed enough cognitive reserve to handle unexpected challenges. The long-term effects of brain injuries are unpredictable;
some days are better than others. I needed to know that on a bad day,
I could still manage the basics: take my medication correctly, recognize if something was wrong, ask for help if I needed it.

But I also wrote down what I was willing to sacrifice:

I was willing to accept that I would never be able to work full-
time again. The 40-hour work week, the career ladder, the professional ambitions I'd had before the injury, I had to let that go. Was I
ok with doing this? Did I have a choice?

I was willing to have fewer social obligations. The extended
family get-togethers, the constant need to stay busy like my pre-
injury life, I could live without them if it meant having more energy
for what truly mattered.

I was willing to accept some level of seizure risk if it meant a
better quality of life. The illusion of perfect seizure control at the cost
of being unable to think clearly or connect with people I loved wasn't
actually 'better', it was just a different kind of diminished existence.

This exercise, writing down both what I needed and what I was
willing to sacrifice, clarified something crucial: Healthcare tradeoffs
are inevitable. You can't optimize for everything simultaneously. The
question isn't whether you'll make sacrifices, it's which sacrifices you
can live with and which ones you can't.

When I discussed my thought with my neurologist's I felt our
relationship had changed. We were talking about my unattainable
pursuit of being seizure free, but what did I want my life to hopefully
look like. We discussed what was important to me in the short-term
and also my long-term goals. Since then we talk about my desire to

write, to engage with family, to maintain the cognitive functions I'd identified as non-negotiable. He also let me appreciate that there is no certainty with a seizure disorder.

Did these goals change my seizure frequency? No. I still struggle with cognitive clarity however I can write again. I can mostly follow conversations without that frustrating sense of thoughts slipping away before I could grasp them. I could be present with my family in ways that mattered more than any marginal improvement in seizure control.

Was I 'getting better'? Depends on how you measure. But I was living according to my own priorities instead of someone else's definition of optimal outcomes. And that felt like sovereignty.

Sarah's Wake-Up Call: When Prevention Becomes a Prison

Something had shifted for Sarah. You may remember from Chapter 4 how Sarah used AI tools to organize her health questions and prepare for appointments. It was working brilliantly, until it wasn't. Eventually, that desire for perfect organization turned into a trap. She has Type 2 diabetes, which she's been managing for the last five years. For the first two years after her diagnosis, Sarah was what her endocrinologist, Dr. Cara Webster, called 'the gold standard patient.' She tracked her continuous glucose monitor religiously. She logged every meal in her nutrition app. She exercised six days a week—cardio and strength training, carefully planned and executed. Her fasting glucose had dropped from 104 to 92. Her blood pressure was textbook perfect. By every clinical measure, her prevention strategy was working brilliantly.

But Sarah was miserable.

The breaking point came on a Saturday morning. She'd just finished her scheduled workout, 40 minutes of interval training, logged and analyzed, when her best friend texted asking if she wanted to grab coffee and pastries at their favorite bakery, just the two of them.

Sarah's immediate response was to calculate whether pastries fit her macro targets for the day. She mentally reviewed her continuous glucose monitor data from the last time she'd eaten refined carbs at breakfast. She started formulating a response about how they could go for a walk afterward to manage the blood sugar spike.

Then she caught herself. And something shifted.

'Let me grab my purse,' she texted back.

At the bakery, watching her friend's face light up over shared stories and laughter, Sarah felt something she hadn't felt in two years of perfect health optimization: joy. Uncomplicated, unquantified joy.

Her continuous glucose monitor showed a spike after the pastry. Her nutrition app flagged that she'd exceeded her carb limit. None of it mattered in that moment.

That night, Sarah started her own version of the list I'd made. Not what she should want for her health, but what she actually wanted for her life:

She wanted to prevent the serious complications her grandmother had experienced from diabetes. That was real and non-negotiable.

But she also wanted spontaneous coffee dates with her friends. She wanted to be able to accept dinner invitations without mentally calculating macros. She wanted to exercise because it felt good, not because her metrics demanded it. She wanted health practices that enhanced her life rather than ones that became her life.

When Sarah discussed her realization with Dr. Webster, she expected resistance. Instead, her doctor nodded with recognition. 'You're not the first patient I've seen become so rigid about prevention that they forget why they're preventing anything in the first place,' she said. 'The goal isn't to live as long as possible while being miserable. It's to have as many good years as possible.'

Together, they redefined Sarah's prevention strategy. She kept the practices that felt sustainable and life-enhancing: regular exercise that she genuinely enjoyed, a generally healthy eating pattern that allowed flexibility, and regular check-ins with Dr. Webster. But she let go of the exhausting vigilance: the continuous glucose monitoring that had become an obsession, the obsessive meal tracking, the self-imposed rules about 'acceptable' foods.

Her clinical markers are slightly less perfect now. Her fasting glucose hovers around 95 instead of 92. She probably exercises four or five days a week instead of six. And she's consistently happier, more connected with her friends, more present in her life.

When talking about this shift, Sarah puts it simply: 'I realized I was trying to prevent complications by not really living. That's not prevention. That's just a different kind of dying, slower and more organized, but still dying.'

Julie's Metric Treadmill: When Optimization Becomes Obsession

Julie's relationship with her health data had taken a different turn. After years of chronic pain for the past five years. When she first started working with her pain management specialist, Dr. Leo Park, she did what made sense at the time: she tried to track and optimize everything to figure out what reduced her pain.

She tracked everything: which positions made things worse, which exercises helped, which foods seemed to affect inflammation, sleep quality, stress levels, and medication timing. She had spreadsheets. She could tell you her worst days, her best days, her pain patterns by time of day and day of week. She was approaching her chronic pain like a complex puzzle she could solve if she just gathered enough data. It became an obsession.

And for a while, the tracking did help. She identified patterns and felt she was gaining control. She learned that her pain was worse when she skipped sleep or had high-stress weeks. She discovered that certain movements made things better and others worse. Armed with that information, she started optimizing. Better sleep schedule, stress reduction practices, and specific exercises prescribed by a physical therapist. The pain did improve, actually.

But then something shifted. The tracking, which had been a tool, became a burden. Julie found herself anxious on any day that didn't fit the pattern. If she had a bad pain day when she'd 'done everything right,' she experienced it not just as physical pain but as personal failure. She became hyper-vigilant about every variable she'd identified. She was measuring her pain multiple times a day, comparing it to her historical baseline, analyzing whether that half-point increase on the pain scale meant something was wrong.

Her kids started noticing. One day, her teenager said something that stopped her cold: 'Mom, you spend more time with your phone tracking things than you spend with us.'

The comment bothered Julie more than she wanted to admit. That night, after her kids were in bed, she looked at her tracking app. Years of data. Thousands of entries. Countless hours of analysis.

What had it actually gotten her?

She was objectively more knowledgeable about her pain patterns. She had better management strategies. But she was also more anxious, more obsessed with pain metrics, more likely to interpret any deviation as a sign that her condition was getting worse. The tracking had made her quantitatively better but qualitatively miserable.

When Julie brought this up at her next appointment with Dr. Park, she expected him to reassure her that the tracking was helping. Instead, he took her concerns seriously. 'Sometimes measurement becomes the disease instead of helping you manage it,' he said. 'The question isn't whether you have good data. It's whether the tracking is serving your actual life.'

After a difficult conversation with Dr. Park, Julie made a decision: she stopped tracking everything. Not completely, but she simplified dramatically. She kept a simple note about particularly bad pain days and what she'd done that day, so she could still notice patterns. But she let go of the spreadsheets, the multiple daily measurements, the constant analysis.

The first week was disorienting. She didn't have her app telling her if her pain was better or worse than yesterday. She had to rely on her own sense of her body instead of comparing to quantitative baselines. She felt untethered.

But gradually, something shifted. She started noticing how she actually felt instead of what her app told her she should feel. She noticed when her body felt better and responded by doing the things that helped, without needing to verify it with data first. She exercised when it felt good, not according to her tracking schedule. She let herself rest when she needed to without worrying that a rest day would show up as a metric failure.

Three months after Julie stopped tracking every pain metric, something shifted. She found herself sitting on the floor playing a board game with her teenagers on a Tuesday evening—something she would have skipped before, worried that sitting cross-legged would trigger a pain spike she'd need to document and analyze.

Her teenager won the game and threw his arms around her in celebration. Julie realized she hadn't checked her pain level once that evening. She hadn't opened her tracking app. She hadn't made mental notes about whether this position or that movement made things worse.

The pain was still there—it was always there. But she'd stopped measuring it incessantly, and in doing so, she'd discovered something unexpected: the constant tracking had become its own kind of pain behavior. The vigilance itself had been exhausting her as much as the chronic pain.

Her pain levels might be slightly higher now by the numbers, if she were still measuring them. But she was present with her family in a way she hadn't been in years. And wasn't that supposed to be the point?

Julie's story illustrates an important truth: What matters to you might be the opposite of what optimization culture tells you should matter. For some people, detailed tracking is empowering, it provides useful data and a sense of control. For others, like Julie, it becomes a prison. Neither approach is objectively right or wrong. The question is what serves your actual life, not what serves some abstract ideal of optimal health.

Mary's Choice: When Your Health Decision Isn't Just About You

The framework of defining what matters isn't just for managing your own health. Sometimes it becomes crucial when your healthcare decisions affect not just you but the people who depend on you.

Mary is a working professional and a caregiver for her mother, who was diagnosed with early-stage Alzheimer's five years ago. Two years into the caregiving journey, Mary was diagnosed with a chronic health condition. Her doctor, Dr. Susan Chang, presented treatment options that both made sense medically but felt impossible emotionally.

Option one: medication management. They would start treatment to control her condition, which would require regular follow-up appointments—monthly at first, then every few months once stabilized—along with periodic lab work to monitor how she was responding. It meant committing to ongoing medical appointments for the foreseeable future.

Option two: surgery. A procedure that could potentially resolve or significantly improve her condition, possibly reducing her need for long-term medication. But surgery meant recuperation—weeks of recovery when she wouldn't be able to care for her mother. It also carried surgical risks and the possibility of complications that could extend her recovery even longer.

'What would you recommend?' Mary asked, her voice quieter than she intended.

Dr. Chang paused, choosing her words carefully. 'Medically, both are reasonable options. Surgery might give you a better long-term outcome. But I can't make this decision without understanding what's happening in the rest of your life. What else are you managing right now?'

Mary told her about her mother. About how the Alzheimer's was progressing, how her mother needed help with daily tasks now, how Mary had already reduced her work hours to be there. About how her mother still recognized her, still lit up when Mary walked in the room, but that window was closing. Maybe a year, maybe two, before her mother wouldn't know who she was anymore.

Dr. Chang listened, really listened. Then she said something Mary hadn't expected: 'These aren't just medical decisions. They're life decisions. And you're the only one who can weigh what matters most right now.'

Mary went home and sat with her mother that evening. They watched old photos together, her mother pointing at pictures and sometimes remembering the stories, sometimes not. Mary held her mother's hand—a hand that had held hers through childhood, through hard times, through everything. And she knew.

She got out a notebook later that night and worked through the questions.

What does a good day look like? For Mary, it meant being present for these afternoons with her mother. It meant being there when her mother got confused and needed reassurance. It meant having these precious ordinary moments—folding laundry together, watching game shows, just sitting quietly side by side. Time she could never get back once it was gone.

What was she willing to sacrifice? Mary was willing to commit to regular medical appointments if it meant she could keep showing up for her mother every day. She was willing to take medication long-term. She was willing to accept that this wasn't the medically optimal choice for her own health outcomes.

What was she not willing to sacrifice? She couldn't give up these months or years with her mother while her mother still knew her. Surgery meant six to eight weeks of recovery, maybe longer if there were complications. That was time Mary couldn't get back. Her mother's decline wouldn't pause while Mary healed.

Who was she optimizing for? This was the question that made everything clear. She could optimize for her own health by choosing surgery. It made sense medically. But she would be choosing her own long-term health over her mother's immediate need for her presence. In another season of life, surgery might be the obvious choice. But not now. Not during this small, closing window when her mother still recognized her daughter's face.

Mary chose medication management. When she told Dr. Chang, she expected judgment or disappointment. Instead, her doctor nodded with understanding.

'We'll monitor you carefully,' Dr. Chang said. 'Monthly appointments for the first few months, then we'll see how you're responding. Yes, it's more appointments than surgery would have been long-term. But it means you can be there for your mother now, during this time that matters so much to both of you. That's not a failure of decision-making. That's wisdom.'

Mary's treatment plan looks different from what might be medically optimal for her condition alone. She takes her medication daily. She shows up for her appointments, sometimes bringing her mother with her when she can't find other care. She manages the logistics of ongoing medical management. But every afternoon, she's sitting with her mother. Every evening, she's there. She's present for this season of life that won't come again.

Her choice shows something profound: The framework of defining what matters isn't selfish. Sometimes the most important healthcare decision is recognizing that your health exists in relationship to other people's wellbeing. Sometimes the sovereign choice is the one that lets you be present for the people you love, even if it's not the choice that optimizes your own medical outcomes. Sometimes choosing love over optimal health is the wisest medical decision you can make.

The Three Questions That Clarify Everything

After working through my own priority-defining process and hearing similar stories from other patients, I've distilled the work of figuring out what matters into three core questions. These questions have helped me make every significant healthcare decision since my brain injury, and I've shared them with countless other patients who've found them equally clarifying.

These aren't questions you answer once and forget. They're questions you return to regularly, especially when facing new treatment decisions, when your health status changes, or when you notice your healthcare isn't actually supporting the life you want to live.

Question 1: What Does a Good Day Look Like?

Not a perfect day. Not an ideal day if you had unlimited health and energy. A good day, a day where you'd go to bed thinking I was successful. It might just be the ability to do one simple stretching exercise or enjoying a long walk with my service dog Gabe.

For me right now, a good day starts with waking up and actually knowing it's morning, not that disoriented fog where I'm not sure if I slept or what day it is. It includes making coffee and tasting it properly, not through the metallic filter that some medications create. It includes opening my laptop and being able to hold a thought long enough to get it into words, then another thought, then another, until I've written something that makes sense. It includes at least one meaningful conversation with someone I care about where I'm fully present. It includes basic self-care tasks without exhausting myself.

In the first year after the medication dosage mistake, a good day looked completely different. Back then, it meant being able to walk around the house with my walker without collapsing. It meant showering without needing to lie down afterward, exhausted from the effort of basic hygiene. It meant watching a TV show and actually following the plot instead of staring blankly at moving images. The bar wasn't quality of life—it was survival and basic function.

Now, almost four years later, my definition has evolved. I've adapted to my new baseline. I know I'll never have the cognitive endurance I used to have, so I've stopped measuring good days against that impossible standard from the past. Instead, I measure against what's actually possible now.

This clarity matters because it gives you a way to evaluate treatment tradeoffs. If a medication eliminates your symptoms but leaves you so fatigued you can't do the things that make a good day good, is it actually helping? If a treatment plan technically improves your clinical markers but requires so much time and energy that you can't have good days, is it worth it? These are tough discussions you need to have with your provider.

Your good day will be different from mine. Maybe it's being able to exercise without pain. Maybe it's having energy to play with your kids after work. Maybe it's being able to cook dinner instead of ordering in. Maybe it's being able to focus on complex work tasks. Maybe it's something that has nothing to do with productivity at all—just enjoying your morning coffee without anxiety, or having a day without migraines, or being able to sleep through the night.

The point is to get specific about what actually brings quality to your days. Not what should matter, not what matters to other people, but what makes your life feel worth living.

Question 2: What Are You Willing to Sacrifice?

This is the harder question. We all want to believe we can have every-thing—perfect health, full function, no limitations, no tradeoffs. But chronic conditions and serious health challenges force choices. The question isn't whether you'll sacrifice something, it's what you're willing to give up and what you're not.

When I was adjusting my seizure medications, I had to get brutally honest about this. I wasn't willing to sacrifice more cognitive clarity; that was non-negotiable. I wasn't willing to sacrifice my connection with my family anymore. But I was willing to sacrifice perfect seizure control, certain social obligations, and some inde-pendence.

One of the most profound losses in chronic illness is rarely discussed in medical appointments: the loss of professional identity. We build our sense of self around what we can do, what we deliver, how we perform. For many people, work isn't just how they earn a living—it's proof of their value, evidence of their competence, the measure by which they know themselves.

Chronic conditions force a reckoning with this identity. The person who prided themselves on high performance finds themselves unable to sustain previous work levels. The professional who never misses deadlines discovers that managing their health requires letting opportunities pass. The individual who defined themselves through career achievement must confront a future that looks nothing like what they'd imagined.

This isn't a simple adjustment. It's grief. Real, deep grief for the professional future that's been foreclosed. The trajectory that will never happen. The version of yourself you'll never become.

Some try to preserve the old identity through sheer force of will—accepting more aggressive medication regimens for better symptom control, structuring their entire lives around work performance, sacrificing relationships, rest, and everything else that gives life meaning. It's understandable. Work feels like what makes us valuable. Letting it go feels like becoming less.

But eventually, if you're paying attention, you realize this approach requires sacrificing what you've decided is non-negotiable. The medication side effects that steal cognitive clarity. The exhaustion that leaves nothing for family. The constant pushing that makes every day feel like survival rather than living.

The paradox is this: Letting go of who you were professionally can become a kind of liberation. Not immediately—first comes the grief, and that grief is legitimate and necessary. But once you stop trying to force yourself back into a shape that no longer fits, space opens for something else. Not better, not what you'd have chosen, but real. A life built around what's actually possible now, rather than what used to be possible then.

This isn't about giving up or accepting defeat. It's about being strategic with limited resources. Every person managing a chronic condition has finite energy, finite capacity, finite reserves. The question becomes: How do you allocate those limited resources to maximize what matters most? Sometimes the answer requires letting go of professional ambitions that, however painful to release, would consume everything you have and leave nothing for the things you've decided you can't sacrifice.

The people who navigate this well don't do it through optimism or determination. They do it through clarity—brutal, honest clarity about what they're optimizing for. And sometimes, after the grief passes, they discover that a smaller professional life creates space for a larger actual life.

Your sacrifices will be personal to you. Maybe you're willing to tolerate side effects that would be unacceptable to someone else because the core benefit matters more to you. Maybe you're willing to have fewer good days if it means avoiding a treatment you find intolerable. Maybe you're willing to sacrifice longevity for quality of the years you have.

There's no right answer to this question, only your answer. And your answer can change as your circumstances change. The key is to know your answer right now, for this decision, given your current life and values.

Question 3: Who Are You Optimizing For?

This question cuts to the heart of sovereignty.

When you make healthcare decisions, whose priorities are you serving? Yours? Your doctor's? Your family's? Your employer's? Society's expectations of what a 'good patient' does?

It's easy to lose yourself in the expectations others have for your health. Your doctor wants optimal clinical outcomes. Your family wants you to be 'back to normal.' Your employer wants you functional enough to work. The wellness industry wants you pursuing constant optimization. Well-meaning friends want you to try whatever worked for someone they know.

All of these stakeholders have opinions about what you should do with your body and your healthcare. And some of their input might be valuable—doctors have medical expertise, family knows you deeply, friends want to help. But ultimately, you're the one living in your body. You're the one experiencing the side effects, managing the limitations, making the daily accommodations. You're the one who has to live with the consequences of every healthcare decision.

The challenge is that these different priorities often conflict. A treatment that optimizes your clinical markers might leave you unable to do the things that make your life feel worth living. A medication that satisfies your family's desire to see you 'back to normal' might require cognitive tradeoffs you find unacceptable. An aggressive protocol that impresses your doctor might be unsustainable given your actual life circumstances.

The best doctors understand something crucial: medical decisions become straightforward once you're clear on your priorities. The complexity isn't in the clinical evidence—it's in determining what you're trying to achieve. If seizure control is your highest priority and you're willing to accept cognitive tradeoffs to get it, certain medications make sense. If maintaining cognitive function matters most and you're willing to accept some symptom risk, different choices emerge. The medical expertise can guide you once you've decided what you're optimizing for. But only you can determine your priorities.

This is what true partnership in healthcare looks like. Not a parent-child dynamic where the doctor decides what's best, but a collaboration where medical expertise serves your priorities. The doctor brings knowledge of what treatments can do. You bring knowledge of what matters in your actual life. Together, you can make decisions that are medically sound and personally meaningful.

The paradox is that what's optimal for you might not be optimal by purely clinical metrics. You might choose a treatment that leaves your numbers less perfect but your life more livable. You might accept more symptoms to preserve the functions that matter most to you. You might prioritize sustainability over aggressiveness, presence over perfection, meaning over metrics.

These aren't failures of medical decision-making. They're evidence that you've gotten clear on who you're optimizing for: yourself, not someone else's version of what your health should look like.

The sovereign patient isn't the one who achieves the best clinical outcomes. It's the one who achieves outcomes that align with what they've decided matters most—even when those decisions puzzle their doctors, disappoint their families, or violate conventional wisdom about optimal care.

Because at the end of the day, you're not trying to be the perfect patient. You're trying to live your life, with all its constraints and priorities and values, while managing a health condition as best you can. And that requires knowing—really knowing—who you're optimizing for and having the courage to make decisions accordingly.

When Your Answers Surprise You

There's a phenomenon I've observed in myself and in other patients working through these questions: Sometimes your answers reveal an uncomfortable gap between what you say matters and what your choices actually reveal.

I said family was my top priority. Connection, presence, relationship, those were what mattered most to me, what I'd identified as non-negotiable.

But when I looked honestly at how I was actually allocating my limited energy the story was different. I was spending my best cognitive hours, the morning time when my brain worked most clearly on other tasks. I was saving social time for evening, when I was depleted and foggy. To this day I still fight this issue.

My stated priorities were social. My revealed priorities were saying something different. For example, if I say my health is a priority then I need to do my exercise first thing in the morning versus putting it off to the end of the day.

This misalignment isn't dishonesty. It's human. We hold multiple, sometimes conflicting values. We want to be the kind of person who prioritizes family over career, who values quality over quantity, who lives according to our deepest values. But we're also afraid of being seen as lazy, or we're clinging to professional identity, or we're avoiding the grief of accepting our limitations.

The value of the three questions isn't just in answering them, it's in comparing your answers to your actual choices and confronting the gaps.

When I recognized that my choices didn't match my stated priorities, I had to do some difficult work. Was I lying to myself about what mattered? Or was I making choices that didn't serve what genuinely mattered because of fear, pride, or external pressure?

I realized it was the latter. Family genuinely mattered most to me. But I was terrified of losing my research identity entirely. I was afraid that if I wasn't productive doing things, I had no value. So I was sabotaging my stated priority to serve my fear.

That recognition allowed me to make different choices. I started protecting my morning cognitive energy for what was most important to me. I saved my depleted evening energy for relaxation and hobby time. These are things that don't require my full brain.

The gap between stated and revealed preferences isn't failure. It tells you either that you need to change your choices to align with your values, or that you need to get more honest about what you actually value versus what you think you should value.

The key is honesty. Your answers to the three questions should match your choices. If they don't, something needs to change, either your answers or your choices. And usually, that change starts with admitting what you're really optimizing for, even if it's not what you wish you were optimizing for.

The Practice of Revisiting What Matters

Here's something crucial about living with chronic conditions: What matters to you isn't static. It changes as your health changes, as your life circumstances evolve, as you adapt to new realities, as your priorities shift.

In the early stages of a chronic condition, many people are willing to sacrifice almost anything for symptom control. The diagnosis is new, the fear is fresh, every symptom feels like a catastrophe. Patients accept severe side effects, aggressive treatments, major life disruptions—anything that promises relief or control. This makes sense. When you're newly diagnosed or experiencing acute crisis, survival and stability are the only priorities that matter.

But over time, the relationship with a condition changes. You learn your patterns, develop management strategies, build confidence in your ability to handle flare-ups or breakthrough symptoms. What once felt catastrophic becomes manageable. And as that relationship shifts, so do your priorities. You might start optimizing for quality of life rather than perfect symptom control. You might accept some level of symptoms to avoid side effects you've decided are worse than the condition itself. You might prioritize energy, cognitive clarity, or presence with loved ones over achieving the best possible clinical markers.

Neither priority set is wrong. They're appropriate for different stages of living with a chronic condition. The person in year one who accepts anything for symptom control isn't making a mistake. The person in year five who prioritizes quality of life over perfect management isn't giving up. They're both responding appropriately to where they are in their journey.

This is why revisiting the three questions regularly matters so much. What does a good day look like now? What are you willing to sacrifice at this stage? Who are you optimizing for with your current treatment approach?

These aren't questions you answer once and file away. They're questions you return to—every six months, annually, whenever something changes significantly in your health or life. Sometimes your answers stay the same. Sometimes they shift subtly. Occasionally they change dramatically, which signals it's time to reconsider your treatment approach.

This practice serves as an early warning system. When you notice your answers centering more and more on external expectations—work productivity, others' opinions, societal definitions of health—rather than your own values, you can catch the drift before it becomes a crisis. When you realize you're sacrificing things you said were non-negotiable, you have information to act on. When your stated priorities no longer match your actual choices, you can investigate the gap.

The people who navigate chronic conditions well over the long term don't do it through rigid adherence to a single approach. They do it through regular reassessment and willingness to adjust. They recognize that managing a chronic condition isn't a problem you solve once—it's a relationship you tend over time, adapting as both you and your condition evolve.

This doesn't mean you're inconsistent or indecisive. It means you're responsive to reality. Your condition changes. Your life circumstances change. Your capacity changes. Your values might shift as you gain experience living with your condition. Rigidly holding to priorities that no longer serve you isn't strength—it's stubbornness. Regularly reassessing and adjusting isn't weakness—it's wisdom.

The framework of defining what matters works because it's dynamic. You're not locked into the priorities you identified when you were first diagnosed. You're empowered to revisit them, revise them, and realign your treatment approach accordingly. That's not just patient empowerment. That's patient sovereignty in practice.

This work never ends. That might sound discouraging, but I find it liberating. I don't have to get the answers perfectly right forever. I just have to get them right enough for now, and then revisit them when things change.

Your Turn: The Values Clarity Exercise

If you're reading this and thinking 'I should do this for my own health situation,' I encourage you to start now. Not tomorrow, not after your next appointment, now.

Get a piece of paper or open a note on your phone. Write down the three questions:

1. What does a good day look like for me?
2. What am I willing to sacrifice, and what am I not?
3. Who am I optimizing for with my current healthcare approach?

Don't overthink your first answers. Write what comes immediately to mind. You can refine later.

Then ask yourself: Is my current healthcare actually supporting what I just wrote down? Are my treatments helping me have more good days as I define them? Am I sacrificing the things I said I could sacrifice, or am I giving up things I said were non-negotiable? Am I pursuing health goals that serve my own priorities, or am I pursuing what I think I should want?

If there's misalignment, if your healthcare isn't actually serving what matters to you, that's not a failure. It's incredibly valuable information. It tells you something needs to change. Maybe it's your treatment approach. Maybe it's your priorities, perhaps what you thought mattered doesn't actually matter in practice. Maybe it's the way you're communicating with your doctor about your goals.

Whatever the misalignment reveals, you now have clarity about it. And clarity is power.

I keep my answers to these questions in a note on my phone. Before every doctor's appointment, I review them. They help me stay grounded in what I'm actually trying to achieve rather than getting swept up in clinical discussions about metrics that might not serve my real priorities.

They've helped me say no to treatments that didn't align with my values, even when doctors strongly recommended them. They've helped me say yes to approaches that made sense for my life, even when they weren't the most aggressive clinical options. They've helped me have productive conversations with my healthcare team about what success actually looks like for me.

Most importantly, they've helped me feel like a sovereign over my own healthcare rather than a subject following orders. Because I'm not pursuing health in the abstract, I'm pursuing my health, defined by my values, in service of my life.

THE FOUNDATION OF EVERYTHING THAT FOLLOWS

This chapter might feel different from the others. It's more introspective, more about internal work than external action. There are no specific AI tools to use, no scripts for doctor conversations, no step-by-step protocols.

That's intentional.

Everything else in this book, asking better questions, building your healthcare team, controlling your data, having transformative conversations with your doctors, all of it rests on this foundation: knowing what matters to you.

You can't effectively advocate for yourself if you don't know what you're advocating for. You can't evaluate treatment options if you don't know what you're optimizing for. You can't be sovereign over your healthcare if you're pursuing someone else's definition of health.

The clarity you develop here enables everything that follows. In Chapter 11, when you're learning to have transformative conversations with your doctors, you'll know what you're trying to communicate and why it matters. In Chapter 12, when you're building your action plan, you'll know what success looks like. The frameworks and tools in later chapters work because they're built on this foundation of knowing what matters.

And here's what I've learned: this work evolves. My definition of what matters has shifted multiple times over my journey with TBI. What mattered in the acute crisis phase was different from what mattered in the adaptation phase, which is different from what matters now in long-term management. My priorities will likely shift again as I age, as my condition changes, as my life circumstances evolve. That's not failure, that's being human with a chronic condition in a changing life.

This clarity work isn't easy. It requires confronting uncomfortable questions about tradeoffs and sacrifices. It requires getting honest about whose expectations you've been serving. It requires the vulnerability of defining what matters to you and the courage to pursue it even when it doesn't align with conventional wisdom or clinical guidelines or others' opinions about what you should want.

But this work is the foundation of patient sovereignty. Without it, all the tools and techniques and communication strategies in the world won't help you get the healthcare that actually serves your life. With it, everything else becomes clearer, more focused, more effective.

You deserve healthcare that serves the life you want to live, not some generic template of optimal health. You deserve to make decisions based on your values, your priorities, your circumstances, not on what works for the average patient or what's easiest for the system or what looks best on paper.

But first, you have to know what that life looks like. You have to define what matters.

So before you move on to the next chapter, before you start planning your next doctor conversation or building your action plan or implementing any of the tools in this book, do the work of this chapter.

Answer the three questions. Write them down. Sit with them. Revise them. Compare them to your actual choices and confront any gaps. Share them with people you trust. Bring them to your next medical appointment.

Because once you're clear on what matters to you, everything else becomes possible.

That's not just patient empowerment. That's patient sovereignty.

The Values Audit

Let's expand on those initial three questions even more. Take time to work through these prompts. Write your answers in a journal or document you can revisit as your health and circumstances change. This might be something you keep to yourself or you may share with someone special in your life.

1. Describe your ideal "good day" with your health condition (not a perfect day, a realistic good day):

2. What would you be doing?

3. Who would you be with?

4. How would you feel?

5. What would be possible?

6. What are you willing to sacrifice to protect what matters most?

7. What are you NOT willing to sacrifice, no matter what?

8. How might your definition of a "good day" change as your health status evolves?

THE CONVERSATION
THAT TRANSFORMS CARE

Chapter 10 was about getting clear on what matters most to you, even when your symptoms, fear, or fatigue try to drown that clarity out. Chapter 11 is about the next step: turning that inner clarity into words your healthcare team can actually use.

From my experience, knowing what you need is powerful, but it only changes your care when you can communicate it in a way that fits the realities of a rushed appointment, a busy clinic, and a record that reduces human lives to checkboxes.

THE BRIDGE FROM KNOWING TO SPEAKING

Julie sat in her car in the hospital parking lot, her hands tracing the edges of the preparation form she'd printed the night before. She had spent weeks doing the internal work from Chapter 10, defining what mattered to her: being mentally present for her two teenagers mattered more than achieving a perfect zero-pain score on some clinical scale. She had clarity about her "Good Day"—one where she could help with homework without pain making her short-tempered, where she could play a board game with her kids without the fog of medication stealing the moment.

But knowing what mattered and communicating it effectively to Dr. Leo Park were two entirely different challenges.

This is the gap that stops most people. You do the internal work. You achieve clarity about your priorities. You feel ready. And then you sit across from your doctor in that sterile exam room, and suddenly you're back in the familiar script: answering their closed-ended questions, nodding along, leaving with a plan you didn't help create.

For years, Julie's appointments with Dr. Park had followed what we discussed in Chapter 1—the Extraction Paradigm. He would ask for her pain level on a scale of one to ten, review her medication logs, order tests, adjust dosages. He was an expert in nerve damage, but he never once asked what mattered to her. It was a cycle of "rinse and repeat" that left Julie feeling sicker and more invisible with every visit.

She was done with the repetition. She didn't just want things to change; she needed them to change.

The transition from sovereign knowledge to sovereign action requires a specific skill: the ability to have transformative conversations with your healthcare providers. This isn't about being difficult or demanding. It's about communicating what you need in a way that invites partnership rather than resistance.

That's what this chapter is about—bridging the gap between knowing what matters and being able to voice it effectively. We're moving from the internal reflection of the previous chapter into the actual dialogue that shifts you from a subject of extraction to a sovereign partner.

Why Medical Conversations Fail

The average primary care visit in the United States lasts eighteen minutes. Within that window, doctors are expected to review your history, perform an exam, order tests, make diagnoses, and document everything in the electronic health record. Research has found that primary care physicians spend an average of eleven seconds on each clinical decision during a typical visit.

Eleven seconds.

It's no wonder conversations feel rushed, transactional, incomplete. But time pressure isn't the only barrier. The structure of medical training itself creates a script that's hard to break.

Medical students learn to conduct interviews using a standardized format: Chief Complaint, History of Present Illness, Past Medical History, Review of Systems. This format is efficient for data extraction, but it turns patients into sources of information rather than people with stories. The questions are closed-ended, the flow is predetermined, and there's little room for what really matters to you.

Then there's the power differential. Your doctor has spent years mastering specialized knowledge. You're sitting there in a paper gown, vulnerable and uncertain. Even with the best intentions, this dynamic makes true partnership difficult. Published analyses confirm that patients speak less than thirty percent of the time during medical visits, and much of that time is spent answering direct questions rather than volunteering information they consider important.

Add to this the electronic health record—that screen your doctor keeps looking at instead of you. It's supposed to improve care, but it often becomes a barrier to eye contact and the kind of attention that makes a person feel heard.

But here's what I've learned: even within these constraints, transformative conversations are possible. They require both parties to show up differently. They require doctors willing to practice a different kind of medicine, and patients willing to claim a different kind of role.

Julie's Turning Point: The Question That Changed Everything

The moment that broke the cycle for Julie didn't happen in Dr. Park's office. It happened when she met her primary care physician, Dr. Susan Chang, for the first time. Before the clinical exam even began, Dr. Chang asked a question that almost made Julie cry:

"What does a good day look like for you?"

Julie's answer was specific. A good day was being able to help her kids with homework without pain making her short-tempered. It was going to the grocery store without having to sit down halfway through the aisles. It was not having to apologize to her family for being grumpy because she was hurting.

Dr. Chang leaned forward. "Okay. That's the definition of 'good' we'll use. We're not aiming for zero pain, because that may not be realistic. We're aiming for the pain level where you can be the mom and person you want to be."

That conversation was Julie's wake-up call. It gave her the "Good Day" metric—a tool more powerful than any clinical scale. But Julie also realized a difficult truth: she couldn't rely on every doctor to be like Dr. Chang. Most of the medical system is still built on extraction. If she wanted her care with Dr. Park to change, she couldn't wait for him to ask the right questions. She had to bring her "Good Day" definition to him.

This brings us back to Julie sitting in her car in the hospital parking lot, preparing to walk into Dr. Park's office and demand a transformative conversation.

The Six Elements of Transformative Conversations

After years of navigating the healthcare system with a chronic condition, I've identified six elements that distinguish transformative conversations from ordinary medical encounters. These elements work together to shift the dynamic from paternalism to partnership.

Element One: Mutual Agenda-Setting

Transformative conversations begin with both parties stating what they hope to accomplish. Julie knew that if she didn't speak first, Dr. Park would fall back into his script. At the very start of the visit, she said:

"I know you want to review my pain logs, and I do too. But I also need to talk about how this medication is making me too foggy to be present with my kids. That's my priority today."

By stating her agenda clearly, she established herself as a partner in the conversation, not just a recipient of care.

Element Two: Full Context Sharing

Medical decisions don't happen in isolation; they happen in the context of your life. Julie moved beyond the clinical checklist to share her full context. She explained that "better" to her meant being able to play a board game with her teenagers on Tuesday nights. This gave Dr. Park information that no pain log would capture—information that proved essential for their treatment decisions.

Element Three: Thinking Out Loud Together

In traditional medical encounters, doctors think privately and then announce conclusions. Julie invited Dr. Park to share his diagnostic reasoning process. When he suggested a dosage adjustment, she asked, "What are the trade-offs you're weighing right now?"

This prompted him to think out loud. He explained that lowering the dose might reduce her cognitive fog but could also allow more breakthrough pain. This transparency shifted Julie from a recipient of orders to a collaborator in the clinical reasoning process.

Element Four: Explicit Uncertainty

One of the most powerful shifts in the visit occurred when Dr. Park acknowledged what medicine often hides: uncertainty. He admitted, "Honestly, Julie, we're not sure what the perfect dose is for your specific nerve sensitivity."

In the past, this might have felt like a lack of expertise. Now, it built trust. Julie understood they were in a collaborative process of discovery, where her daily observations weren't "complaints" but essential data needed to adjust the approach.

Element Five: Decision Ownership

As the appointment drew to a close, they made the ownership of each decision explicit. Dr. Park stated, "The medical recommendation for this specific drug is my responsibility. But the decision of whether the side effects are worth it belongs entirely to you."

He recognized that only Julie could weigh those trade-offs against her "Good Day" metric. This clarity prevented the resentment that arises when ownership is unclear, ensuring Julie felt supported but never forced.

Element Six: Ongoing Dialogue

Finally, they agreed that their transformative conversation wouldn't end when the exam room door closed. They established a commitment to ongoing dialogue through the patient portal. Julie agreed to send a brief summary every two weeks, noting whether her cognitive fog allowed her to stay present for her kids' homework.

This shifted her care from a series of discrete transactions into a continuous relationship, supported by simple tracking tools that kept Dr. Park updated between visits.

Technology enables this kind of continuous conversation in ways that weren't possible before. Secure messaging, patient portals, symptom tracking apps—these tools support the kind of partnership that transforms care. But the technology is just the infrastructure. What matters is the commitment to ongoing dialogue, to treating healthcare as a continuous relationship rather than a series of discrete transactions.

Sarah's Turning Point

Sarah's journey to transformative conversations took a different shape. For years, her visits with her endocrinologist, Dr. Cara Webster, followed a predictable and exhausting pattern. Dr. Webster would review her labs, recommend the same textbook lifestyle changes, and send her on her way. Sarah would nod along, but she often left knowing the plan wouldn't work because it ignored the professional realities of her life as a teacher.

The breaking point came during a particularly demanding semester. The combination of an intense teaching schedule, late-night lesson planning, and the constant background anxiety of managing diabetes left her exhausted. One day, her blood sugar spiked dangerously high. That night, she realized that her relationship with her diabetes management—and her doctor—had to change.

At her next appointment, Sarah used the Six Elements to shift the dynamic. She opened with Mutual Agenda-Setting: "I know you want to check my labs, but I also want to talk about why I keep saying I'll make these lifestyle changes and then don't. I want to figure out what's actually realistic for me."

Dr. Webster paused and listened as Sarah shared her Full Context. Sarah explained that she often skipped breakfast because she was rushing to her early morning classes and would grab whatever food was quick and easy when she was grading late into the evening.

Instead of a lecture on willpower, they began Thinking Out Loud Together. Dr. Webster said, "You don't need motivation. You need a plan that works with your actual professional schedule." They designed a new approach that included prepping protein-rich snacks on Sundays and eating a handful of nuts before her coffee to stabilize her blood sugar before the school day began.

Three months later, Sarah reflected on the shift: "My A1C is trending in the right direction. But more importantly, I don't feel like a failure anymore. I'm finally managing my diabetes instead of my diabetes managing me."

Caregiving as a Conversation

Mary's story shows how transformative conversations work when you're managing not just your own health, but caregiving responsibilities as well. She's a fifty-eight-year-old marketing manager who balances a high-pressure career with her role as the primary caregiver for her mother, who was diagnosed with early-stage Alzheimer's disease five years ago.

For years, Mary's own healthcare conversations were entirely one-sided. Her doctors would give her standard health recommendations that ignored the reality of her life: she was sleep-deprived, constantly stressed, and had almost no time for herself.

Everything shifted when Mary began seeing Dr. Susan Chang, her primary care physician. At their first appointment, before diving into the clinical data, Dr. Chang asked a question that caught Mary off guard: "What's the hardest part of your week?"

Mary took a long breath and told the truth. The evenings were the breaking point. By the time she helped her mother eat, manage her medications, and get to bed, Mary was too exhausted to do anything but collapse. She wasn't exercising or eating well, but she felt she had no choice if she wanted to be there for her mother.

Dr. Chang nodded and set a new foundation for their partnership. "Your health needs to fit into the time you actually have, not the time you wish you had," she said. "Given that reality, what would actually help you feel more like yourself?"

By sharing her Full Context, Mary and Dr. Chang were able to Think Out Loud Together to design a plan that was sustainable rather than "optimal" on paper. They identified thirty minutes in the morning before her mother woke up as Mary's protected time. Instead of an impossible hour-long workout, they designed a fifteen-minute routine Mary could do at home. Instead of a total dietary overhaul, they focused on one meal she could control. Dr. Chang even referred her to a therapist who could meet via telehealth during Mary's lunch break at work.

Six months later, Mary reflected on the shift in her care. "Dr. Chang never made me feel like I was failing at self-care," she said. "She helped me see that within my real constraints, what I'm doing IS self-care. I still have a demanding job and my mom's Alzheimer's to manage, but I don't feel like I'm drowning anymore."

The Practice of Preparation

Transformative conversations rarely happen by accident. They require preparation—not because you're going to read from a script, but because the act of preparing clarifies your thinking and gives you something to ground you when you inevitably get nervous or feel the time pressure of the clinic.

Before any significant appointment, I now spend twenty minutes getting clear on what I want to accomplish, what information I need to share, what questions need to be answered, what decisions need to be made, and what concerns I might be reluctant to voice.

I write this down. Not in perfect sentences, but in fragments and bullet points that capture what matters. When the appointment starts and I feel the familiar pressure to just answer questions and get out, I have this written anchor to remind me of my actual agenda.

I've also learned to be direct about what I need from the conversation. "I'm feeling overwhelmed and need you to help me prioritize," or "I'm confused about my options and need you to explain them more slowly." These statements aren't rude. They're collaborative. They help your doctor understand how to partner with you effectively.

To make this preparation systematic, I use a simple framework. Before my next appointment, I spend fifteen minutes thinking through these prompts:

- What is the most important thing I want to discuss at this appointment?

- What information does my doctor need to know about my life right now?
- What am I worried or anxious about?
- What specific questions do I have?
- What side effects or concerns am I experiencing?
- What's one thing that's going well that I want my doctor to know about?
- What do I need from this conversation—more time, clearer explanations, a partnership approach?

This preparation doesn't guarantee a transformative conversation. But it dramatically increases the odds that you'll leave the appointment having discussed what actually matters to you, not just what the standard protocol covers.

One Practical Technique: Teach-Back

There's a simple technique that bridges the gap between expert explanation and patient understanding. Medical educators call it "Teach-Back." After explaining something complex—a new medication schedule, the trade-offs of a treatment plan—the doctor asks, "Can you tell me in your own words what we just discussed?"

It's vital to remember that this isn't a test of your memory or intelligence. It's quality control for the doctor's communication. If you can't explain the plan back clearly, the doctor knows they need to explain it differently until your partnership is based on shared understanding rather than just polite nodding.

I've learned to prompt this technique even when my doctor doesn't. At the end of important conversations, I summarize what we've decided: "Let me make sure I understood correctly. We're lowering the dose to prioritize cognitive function, even if it means some breakthrough symptoms, and I'll message you in two weeks with an update."

By initiating the teach-back myself, I ensure we're leaving the room with the same roadmap.

The Conversation After the Conversation

One of the most valuable practices I've developed is what I call the conversation after the conversation. This happens in the hour immediately following an important medical appointment.

I used to leave appointments in a fog. Too much information. Too many decisions. Important details I meant to ask about but forgot. Recommendations I thought I understood but didn't. I would get home and realize I couldn't clearly explain to my partner what the doctor had said or what we had decided.

Now I have a system. Within one hour of leaving any significant appointment, I sit in my car or a nearby coffee shop and record a voice memo. I talk through everything that was discussed, every decision that was made, every question I wish I had asked, every point of confusion. Just five minutes of speaking into my phone.

Then I use an AI tool to transcribe and process that voice memo. The AI helps me identify any inconsistencies or gaps in my understanding. It flags medical terms I used incorrectly, which tells me I misunderstood something and need to follow up. It highlights decisions that were made without clear ownership. It catches things I heard wrong or understood wrong while it's still fresh enough to correct.

This process has caught countless potential problems. When I've shared this practice with other patients, many have adopted it. One friend dealing with a complex condition said it transformed her experience: "I realized I was retaining maybe thirty percent of what was said in appointments because I was so overwhelmed. Now I capture everything. My voice memo becomes my external memory."

A vital boundary must be respected: you are not allowed to record your appointments without your provider's consent. This is a legal and ethical boundary you should never violate. The "conversation after the conversation" is your personal reflection, recorded immediately after you leave the exam room, ensuring your voice remains the sovereign authority over your journey.

Technology as Support, Not Replacement

This is where the technology we've been discussing throughout this book becomes crucial. AI tools can support transformative conversations in several powerful ways.

First, they can help you prepare. Before appointments, I use an AI tool to review my symptom tracking data and identify patterns. "What should I make sure to mention?" I ask. The AI might flag that my sleep quality has declined over the past month, or that certain triggers seem to be emerging. This preparation ensures I bring the right information to the conversation.

Second, AI can help translate between medical and plain language. When my doctor uses a term I don't understand, I make a note and look it up immediately afterward using an AI tool that can explain it in context. This helps me stay oriented in complex discussions.

Third, AI can support the ongoing dialogue between appointments. The symptom tracking and automated summaries I send my doctors are generated with AI assistance. I input the raw data; AI identifies patterns and generates a concise update. This makes continuous communication feasible without overwhelming either of us.

But here's the crucial point: AI supports the conversation but doesn't replace it. The technology handles information management, pattern recognition, and routine communication. The human conversation handles meaning-making, value clarification, and collaborative decision-making. Both are necessary. Neither is sufficient alone.

When Conversations Break Down

Not every attempt at transformative conversation succeeds. Sometimes you encounter a doctor who isn't interested in partnership, who insists on the traditional paternalistic model. Sometimes you're too overwhelmed or unwell to advocate effectively for yourself. Sometimes the system constraints make real dialogue nearly impossible.

I know this from experience. Some of my previous healthcare providers were not interested in the kind of partnership I was seeking. One told me explicitly, "I'm the expert here. Your job is to follow my recommendations." Another was so rushed that every attempt to discuss my concerns was cut off mid-sentence. A third was kind but fundamentally paternalistic—he wanted what was best for me but never asked what I thought was best for me.

When I tried to use the techniques from this chapter with a doctor who wasn't interested in partnership, it didn't matter how well I'd prepared or how clearly I'd stated my agenda. Communication skills aren't enough when one party is fundamentally unwilling to engage in partnership.

When conversations consistently break down, you have three choices. First, you can try to teach your doctor how you need to communicate. This sometimes works, especially with doctors who are well-intentioned but not trained in patient-centered communication. Second, you can work within the constraints by using other resources to fill the gaps—a patient navigator, a support group, other specialists who are more collaborative. Third, you can find a new doctor.

That third option isn't always possible due to insurance, location, or specialty shortages. But when it is possible, it can be transformative. The difference between a doctor who sees you as a partner and one who sees you as a subject of care isn't subtle. It shapes your entire experience of your condition.

From Subject to Partner

The shift from subject to partner in medical care doesn't happen in a single conversation. It's a gradual transformation, built through many small moments of practicing a different way of being in the healthcare system.

Each time you clearly state your agenda at the beginning of an appointment, you're practicing partnership. Each time you ask your doctor to explain their reasoning, you're claiming your right to understand. Each time you share the full context of your life rather than just answering the clinical questions, you're insisting on being seen as a whole person. Each time you say "I need to think about this before agreeing to a treatment," you're exercising your sovereignty.

These small acts accumulate. They reshape your relationship with your healthcare providers. They change how you see yourself—from passive patient to active agent. And remarkably, they often change how your doctors see you too.

Making This Real

You've now completed the critical transition from internal clarity to external articulation. Chapter 10 gave you the tools to define what matters to you: your priorities, your values, your non-negotiables. This chapter has shown you how to communicate that clarity effectively to your healthcare providers, transforming your role from passive subject to active partner.

But transformative conversations don't happen by accident. They require preparation, practice, and systems to support them. Try this before your next appointment: Choose one element from the six we discussed. Just one. Practice it. See what happens. Then come back and add another.

This is how transformation happens—not in grand gestures, but in small, repeated acts of showing up differently until showing up differently becomes who you are.

In the next chapter, we'll move from principle to practice. You'll get specific, actionable tools for systematically implementing patient sovereignty in your ongoing care. We'll build the infrastructure that makes transformative conversations the norm rather than the exception. Understanding that you should be a partner in your care is important. But knowing exactly how to prepare for your next appointment, what questions to ask, how to track your symptoms, when to escalate concerns, and how to maintain ongoing dialogue— that's what makes the difference between theoretical sovereignty and actual agency.

12

YOUR PATIENT ACTION PLAN

In previous chapters, we explored what patient power means. We discussed knowing what matters to you. We talked about speaking clearly with doctors. We covered your right to partner in your own care. Now we move from learning to doing. From ideas to reality. From "someday" to "right now."

This is the operating system for patient power in a system built for patients who just listen.

Everything here is what I have learned managing my own chronic condition. I am not telling you there is one perfect way. That would require perfect organization and unlimited time. I am sharing what actually works in real life. I work with real limits. I manage a chronic medical condition. I maintain relationships. I write when I can. I sometimes have seizures that affect my brain for a few days.

If I can build systems that work even with memory issues and unpredictable symptoms, you can adapt these approaches for your health challenges.

The Foundation: Your Health Dashboard

Everything in this chapter rests on one basic idea: you need one place where all your health information lives. It needs to be organized. It needs to be accessible when you need it. This is not your doctor's system. That system was built for doctors, not for patients. It is often hard to access when you need it most. Your health dashboard is your system. You design it for your needs. You can access it anytime.

I use several tools: a secure note app with AI, a symptom-tracking app, a simple spreadsheet for medications, and folders for test results. The specific tools do not matter as much as the basic ideas. Your dashboard does not need to be electronic. It can be a three-ring binder or even a notebook where you store your tests.

Accessibility: You can access it anywhere, anytime, from any device. My wife and I needed my health information everywhere. We needed it at the testing center when they could not find my blood work. We needed it at my desk while reviewing results. We needed it during a telehealth visit with my specialist. We needed it when scheduling appointments. We needed it on vacation when a new symptom appeared. Cloud-based tools can help make this possible. Just keep your information safe with passwords and encryption.

Completeness: It includes everything relevant to your health. Include current medications and diagnoses. Include past treatments that did not work. Include allergies and bad reactions. Include family health history. Include strategies that worked. Include questions you need to ask. Include decisions you are facing.

Maintainability: It must be simple enough that you will actually keep it updated. Complex systems fail because they are too much work. My health dashboard takes about ten minutes a week to update. I spend time daily updating my symptoms and trends.

Sharing: You can easily share parts of it with your doctors. This means creating exports, PDFs, or printouts that your doctors can use. A simple note can work. But know that it is hard to share. Some doctors cannot upload your information into their system. However, they can view your reports. Talk with your provider to learn what works best for them.

Privacy: Your health information is sensitive. Your dashboard needs security. Use at least password protection. Even better is encryption. I use tools with end-to-end encryption and two-factor authentication. Google Drive and Dropbox also offer this level of protection.

When I first built my health dashboard, I made it too complex. I tried to track everything. I tracked every symptom, every meal, every moment of stress, every medication dose. Within a week I was overwhelmed. I stopped using it. I learned that the perfect system you do not use is worse than the imperfect system you actually use.

My dashboard now tracks only what matters for my conditions. For epilepsy, that means seizure frequency and what they are like. It means medication doses and times. It means sleep quality. It means major stressors. It means how well my brain works. I do not track my diet or exercise unless they affect my seizures, which they haven't. This focused approach makes it sustainable.

The Power of Longitudinal Knowledge

When I first started carefully documenting my health information, it felt like I was just making better records. But over time, I realized I was building something more valuable. I was building knowledge about my own body.

Healthcare systems have institutional knowledge. They see patterns across thousands of patients. They have protocols that have been refined over years. They have clinical guidelines based on data. But they often lack deep knowledge about you specifically. Your medical records capture snapshots. They show what happened at each visit. They show what tests were ordered. They show what was prescribed. They rarely capture the connections between snapshots. They rarely show the patterns that emerge over months or years. They rarely capture the context that shaped each decision.

Your careful documentation creates that missing layer. It is your institutional knowledge about yourself.

After several years of tracking, I can now see patterns that would be invisible in standard medical records. I know which medication changes led to better brain function. I know which environmental factors correlate with seizure clusters. I know how my symptoms evolve across different life circumstances. This long-term perspective makes me a more valuable partner to my doctors. I bring data and insights they cannot get any other way.

A 2024 Cleveland Clinic study examined this. Researchers tracked two groups of patients with chronic conditions over one year. One group received standard care. The other group learned systematic documentation and integration practices.

The results were striking. At 30 days after appointments, the documentation group accurately recalled 73% of their treatment plan details. The standard care group recalled only 38%. At 90 days, the gap widened even further. More importantly, the documentation group had 35% better treatment adherence. They had fewer miscommunications with their care teams. They reported significantly higher confidence in managing their conditions.

The researchers concluded that systematic integration creates a growing advantage. Each documented appointment makes the next appointment more productive. You bring better context. You ask better questions. You spot patterns more readily.

THE SCIENCE OF PREPARATION

Before I share my specific preparation protocol, it helps to understand why preparation matters so much. The research on this is compelling and somewhat concerning.

This is not because we are not paying attention or do not care. It is because of how human memory works under stress. During medical appointments, you feel worried about your health. You are in an unfamiliar environment. You hear complex information with terminology you may not understand. These conditions are precisely the ones where memory fails us most.

But here is the encouraging part: preparation dramatically improves these outcomes. A 2005 study published in Health Communication found that patients who prepared for appointments by writing down their questions in advance had significantly better information recall. They asked more relevant questions. They reported higher satisfaction with their care. The simple act of preparation primed their brains to encode information more effectively.

More recently, a 2024 Johns Hopkins study tracked patients with chronic conditions who used structured appointment preparation tools compared to those who did not. The prepared group had 28% better treatment adherence over the following three months. They had fewer emergency department visits. They reported feeling more confident in managing their conditions. The researchers concluded that preparation provides structure. It helps patients process, retain, and act on medical information.

When I learned about this research, my own preparation habits suddenly made more sense. I was not just being thorough. I was literally changing how my brain processed and retained information from my appointments. I was creating conditions for partnership rather than passive reception.

Preparation: The Pre-Appointment Protocol

The single most powerful thing you can do to transform your medical appointments is to prepare systematically. Do not just think about what you want to discuss. Actually prepare using a structured approach.

Here is the pre-appointment protocol I have developed through trial and error over dozens of appointments.

72 Hours Before: The Information Gather

Three days before any significant appointment, I do a complete review of my health dashboard. I am looking for changes since the last appointment. New symptoms? Medication effects? Life circumstances? I look for patterns in my symptom tracking data. Questions that have emerged. Decisions that need to be made. Test results or records the doctor might not have.

I use an AI assistant to help me organize my symptom tracking and spot possible patterns. I upload my logs and ask: "What trends do you notice over time, and what should I bring to my doctor?" It can help surface signals. A cluster of events during high-stress weeks. Changes after a medication adjustment. A side effect that has been gradually getting worse. I treat these as ideas to discuss, not conclusions.

This is not about replacing medical judgment with AI. It is about using AI as a pattern-recognition tool. I analyze my own data. I have found that AI-assisted summaries based on systematic tracking are more useful than relying on memory. Memory is notoriously unreliable for complex medical information.

A 2024 Harvard Medical School pilot study examined this exact practice. Patients using AI assistants for appointment preparation versus those who did not. The AI-assisted group asked 40% more clinically relevant questions during appointments. They brought up 60% more previously unmentioned symptoms that proved important for diagnosis. They reported significantly higher confidence in their ability to participate in treatment decisions. The researchers noted that AI did not replace clinical judgment. It enabled patients to bring better-organized, more complete information to their clinical encounters.

I want to be clear: the AI is just a tool, not an all-seeing oracle. I do not ask it to diagnose my conditions or recommend treatments. I use it to analyze my own data. I identify patterns worth discussing. I prepare questions worth asking. The actual medical reasoning still happens in partnership with my healthcare providers. They have the clinical expertise. They know my full history. They can examine me. No AI possesses these abilities.

24 Hours Before: The Priority Setting

The day before the appointment, I get clear on my priorities. Medical appointments have limited time. You cannot address everything. What matters most right now?

I write down my top three priorities for the visit, in order. For example: One, discuss increasing brain fog and whether medication adjustment is needed. Two, review recent seizure pattern and what it might show. Three, talk about upcoming work travel and how to manage medication timing.

I also identify my "if there is time" items. These are things I want to address but that are not urgent. Having this clarity prevents me from burying the most important issues under less critical concerns.

This prioritization is harder than it sounds. Everything feels urgent when it is your health. I have learned to ask myself: If I could only address one thing in this appointment, what would it be? That becomes priority one. Then I repeat the question for what is left. This forces genuine prioritization rather than wishful thinking that we will cover everything.

Two Hours Before: The Documentation Prep

A couple of hours before the appointment, I prepare the materials I might need to share. A one-page summary of current symptoms and concerns. Relevant portions of my medical history, labs, and symptom tracking data, formatted clearly. List of current medications with doses. I want to make sure to ask any questions. Any test results or records from other providers.

I print these or have them ready on my phone. If I am doing a telehealth visit, I organize them in a folder on my desktop so I can share my screen if needed.

This preparation typically takes thirty to forty-five minutes total across the three time points. It is the best forty-five minutes I spend on my healthcare. It transforms me from a passive responder to the doctor's questions into an active partner. I bring valuable data and clear priorities.

I know that forty-five minutes of preparation might seem like a lot. But consider the alternative. You show up unprepared. You forget to mention important symptoms. You do not get your questions answered. You leave confused about the plan. You need follow-up appointments to address what you should have covered the first time. The preparation saves time overall.

During the Appointment: Your Participation Framework

How you show up during the appointment matters enormously. Here is the framework I use to maximize the value of every medical conversation.

Opening: State Your Agenda

After initial pleasantries, I immediately and clearly state my agenda. "I know you want to review my test results, and I do too. I also need to discuss these three things today, with the medication side effects being my top priority. Can we make sure we cover all of that?" I tend to overshare, so I have to be very careful to only share the few actionable things the doctor can help me address.

This sets the tone for partnership. It ensures your priorities are on the table from the start. It helps your doctor structure the visit. Most doctors appreciate this clarity. They would rather know upfront what you need than discover it in the last thirty seconds of the appointment.

Middle: Active Listening and Participation

During the discussion, I practice what I call active partnering. I take notes, either on paper or typed on my phone. I ask for clarification immediately when I do not understand something. "Can you explain what you mean by that?" I repeat back key points to confirm understanding. "So you are saying the test results show X, which means Y, and you recommend Z?"

I share my observations and data. "I have been tracking that symptom, and here is what I have noticed." I ask about the reasoning behind recommendations. "Help me understand why you are recommending this approach over alternatives." I voice concerns or disagreements directly. "I am worried about that side effect because..." or "I tried something similar before and it did not work because..."

The goal is genuine dialogue, not interrogation. I am contributing my expertise about my own body and life while learning from my doctor's medical expertise.

Decision Points: Clarify Ownership and Options

When we reach a decision point, I make sure I understand. What exactly are we deciding? What are all the options, including doing nothing? What are the trade-offs of each option? What level of certainty exists about the outcomes? Who owns this decision? Is it me, the doctor, or both of us? What information do I need to make an informed choice? When does the decision need to be made?

I often say explicitly: "Is this my decision to make with your input, your decision to make with my input, or our decision to make together?" That clarity prevents confusion and resentment later.

For significant decisions, I usually say: "I need time to think about this. Can we schedule a follow-up call in a few days after I have processed the information?" Good doctors respect this. Doctors who pressure you to decide immediately are waving a red flag.

Closing: Confirm the Plan

Before the appointment ends, I summarize what we decided and what happens next. "So to confirm: we are going to lower the medication dose from X to Y. I am going to track symptoms for two weeks using the approach we discussed. We will have a follow-up call on this specific date to review how it is going. I will send you my symptom summary three days before that call. Do I have that right?"

This summary serves several purposes. It confirms that we are on the same page. It creates accountability for both of us. It gives the doctor a chance to correct any misunderstandings. And it ensures I leave with a clear action plan, not vague intentions.

I also ask about communication between appointments. "If I notice something concerning before our next appointment, what is the best way to reach you? What symptoms should prompt me to contact you versus wait until our scheduled follow-up?"

After the Appointment: The Integration Process

What you do in the hours after an appointment is almost as important as what you do during it. This is when you integrate what you learned. You update your systems. You use the plan.

My post-appointment protocol has three phases.

Immediately After: Capture Everything

While the appointment is fresh in my mind, I sit in my car or find a quiet spot. I spend ten minutes documenting. Summary of what was discussed. Decisions that were made and the reasoning. New information I learned. Questions that emerged but did not get answered. Action items for me. Action items for the doctor. Follow-up plans.

I often use voice recording for this. I talk through the appointment while it is fresh, then transcribe it later. This captures nuances that note-taking during the appointment might miss.

Within 24 Hours: Update Systems

Within a day of the appointment, I update my health dashboard with new medications or dose changes. I add new diagnoses or updates to existing conditions. I add test results and what they mean. I add changes to my care plan. I schedule the next appointment.

I also update my symptom tracking approach if we decided to monitor different things or in different ways.

Within 48 Hours: Create Action Plan

Within two days, I translate the decisions from the appointment into a concrete action plan. If we decided to try a new medication, my action plan includes when to start. It includes what dose and when to take it. It includes what side effects to watch for. It includes how to track effectiveness. It includes when to follow up. It includes what would trigger earlier contact. It includes questions to research or ask at follow-up.

I set up reminders. I order medications. I schedule follow-up appointments. I configure my tracking tools. I make it as easy as possible for future me to actually use the plan.

This post-appointment process takes about thirty minutes total. It is the difference between leaving an appointment with good intentions and actually implementing the plan. Good intentions fade. Systems work.

Decision-Making Frameworks: From Confusion to Clarity

Medical decisions are hard. They involve uncertainty, trade-offs, technical complexity, and high stakes. Most of us are not trained to make these kinds of decisions. But we can learn frameworks that help.

Here are three frameworks I use for different types of healthcare decisions.

Framework One: The Values-First Approach

For big decisions, I start with values, not medical data. Whether to have surgery. Which medication regimen to try. Whether to participate in a clinical trial. I start with values, not medical data.

I ask myself: What matters most to me in this situation? Common values include maximizing length of life. Maximizing quality of life. Maintaining independence. Minimizing suffering. Being present for important life events. Maintaining cognitive function. Avoiding being a burden on loved ones. Aligning with spiritual or philosophical beliefs. These are big issues involved with many of our healthcare decisions.

I rank these values for this specific decision. Then I evaluate each option against my ranked values. The option that best aligns with what matters most to me is usually the right choice. Even if it is not what the statistics or the doctor would suggest.

For my seizure medication decisions, my top values are maintaining cognitive function. Preventing injury from seizures and falls. Minimizing lifestyle disruption. These values lead me to accept more frequent minor seizures in exchange for less medication and better mental clarity. Someone else with different values, say prioritizing complete seizure control above all else, would make different choices. Both can be right.

Framework Two: The Evidence Hierarchy

When I am trying to evaluate whether a treatment actually works, I use a hierarchy of evidence quality. Highest quality: systematic reviews and meta-analyses of randomized controlled trials. High quality: individual randomized controlled trials. These first two is where you typically will find guidance from your personal doctors. Moderate quality: well-designed observational studies. Lower quality: expert opinion and case studies. Lowest quality: anecdotes and testimonials such as what you might hear from a support group.

I do not dismiss lower-quality evidence. Sometimes it is all we have, and patient experiences matter. But I weigh it appropriately with my healthcare provider. One person's testimonial on a health forum about a miracle supplement is interesting but not convincing. It might even interact with my medications. A systematic review of multiple randomized trials is compelling. Depending on your unique healthcare issue the level of research you decide to explore may be different. You may also be asking how do you do this research. Turning to a respected institution like the Mayo Clinic can be a huge help. They will provide you with expert insights you can trust.

AI tools can be incredibly helpful for navigating this evidence hierarchy. I can ask an AI assistant: "What is the evidence for this treatment approach for my condition? Are there clinical trials? What do systematic reviews say?" The AI can quickly survey the research landscape in ways that would take me hours or days to do manually. Only do this together with your healthcare provider. Remember they are the informed expert on your healthcare situation not an AI tool. I remember my parents turning to reference sources to research a health issue I had, but this alone was not the answer. They would go to our family doctor with what they had read.

Framework Three: The Reversibility Assessment

Some decisions are easily reversible. Others are not. This matters enormously for how to approach them. Also remember I am not a doctor. I am sharing what I have done or considered as a patient. You must talk to your doctor about each of these frameworks.

For highly reversible decisions, like trying a new medication that can be stopped if it does not work, I am willing to experiment with less certainty. "Let us try this for two weeks and see what happens" is a reasonable approach. I have asked my doctor if we start this medication and it is not working or has bad side-effects how difficult is it to stop. This is an important discussion to consider having. Also remember if it involves a medication you must talk to your doctor before making any change.

For irreversible or difficult-to-reverse decisions—like surgery or treatments with permanent side effects—I need much more certainty before proceeding. I will seek second opinions. I do extensive research. I take time to decide.

As I shared above, I explicitly ask my doctors about reversibility: "If we try this and it does not work or causes problems, how easy is it to stop or change course?" The answer shapes if the medication is something I want to explore further.

Communication Systems: Staying Connected Between Appointments

Healthcare does not happen only during appointments. Your symptoms do not pause between visits. Questions emerge. Situations change. Side effects appear. You need systems for communicating with your healthcare team between scheduled appointments.

Here is what I have learned works.

The Regular Update System

I talk to my healthcare providers about how often they would like to communicate with me. For example, every four to six weeks, I send a brief update on how things are going. This is not a novel. It is a structured summary of symptom patterns. Medication adherence and any issues I might be having. Notable symptoms or side effects. Quality of life assessment covering energy, sleep, mood, and cognitive function. Questions or concerns. Anything that needs a response versus just FYI. You can keep this as simple as you like, but just make sure to keep it brief. You do not want to give them anything more to read than what they need. Keep it simple.

I use an AI assistant to help generate these summaries. I input the raw information and AI creates a clear summary in a standard format that I can review. Remember to check these summaries to look for mistakes because AI is not perfect. This takes me about five minutes and it keeps my doctors continuously informed without overwhelming them. Once again I keep this short which might just be a bullet list of no more than ten items.

This regular communication has caught several issues early, before they became crises. It has prevented emergency situations by enabling quick adjustments to treatment plans. A great approach is to also ask your provider if these updates are helping or if I'm oversharing. Some of my doctors like this approach, and to be honest, some read the updates and then never respond. The goal is not to become friends, but to keep them up to date on my healthcare situation.

The Threshold System

I work with my healthcare providers to clearly define thresholds for when I should contact them outside of regular update schedules. We establish categories. Immediate contact by phone for true emergencies. Same-day message for concerning developments. And then things that can wait for regular update for stable patterns and minor questions.

Having these thresholds explicit prevents both under-communicating and over-communicating. I keep them in my health dashboard so I can refer to them when deciding whether something warrants contact.

This will vary based upon your own condition, your medication, and the relationship you have with your provider. For example, I might talk with one of my specialists only once a year. Another I speak to every quarter. Another every six to eight weeks. If you ask them they will tell you what will work best. Just make sure to keep your appointments.

The Documentation Mindset

I rely upon my provider's patient portal for nearly all communications with my healthcare team, not just in-person appointments. When I send an update message, I sometimes will save a copy in my health dashboard. When my doctor responds with guidance, I may save that too. When we have a phone conversation, I write a summary immediately afterward.

This creates a complete record of my care that does not exist anywhere else. My doctor's notes capture their perspective. My documentation captures mine. Both are valuable. The combination is powerful. It is especially powerful when I need to explain my history to a new provider. Or when I need to remember why we made a particular decision months ago.

30-Day Sovereignty Challenge

If you are feeling overwhelmed by all of this, I understand. It is a lot. In fact, at times managing your health can feel like a full-time job, but remember you do not have to use everything at once. In fact, depending upon your healthcare journey, you may not even need some parts of this framework. The most important thing is that you do have a system that works for you. Do not think you need to copy what I have. In fact, you should not try to. Sustainable change happens incrementally as it makes sense to you.

Commit to thirty days of practicing patient sovereignty using some form of this structured approach.

WEEK 1: FOUNDATION

- Create your medical record folder (physical or digital)
- Download your patient portal data and save it on your local computer in a safe and secure location. This information is sometimes called PHI or personal health information.
- Complete the Values Audit from Chapter 10
- List your current medications and why you take each. This is a great thing to keep on your phone. I have had to refer

to this in an emergency room, and I am always so thankful I went through this process ahead of time.

WEEK 2: RELATIONSHIPS

- Use the Question Card from Chapter 7 at your next appointment
- Practice the "Teach-Back" method from Chapter 11
- Identify your healthcare "conductor" role
- Map your care team (who does what?) and share it with someone close to you.

WEEK 3: DATA & PRIVACY

- Review what data you are sharing (apps, devices, portals)
- Anonymize info before using AI tools (Chapter 4 tip). If you need more information about how to do this just ask your favorite AI tool and it will provide some great suggestions.
- Request your full medical records from one provider
- Check your patient portal privacy settings

WEEK 4: ADVOCACY

- Have the "What Matters" conversation from Chapter 11
- Create your personal health narrative (Chapter 6)
- Update your medication list with your observations
- Reflect: What is changed in how you approach your care?

At the end of thirty days, assess what is working. Keep the practices that add value. Modify or discard those that do not. Build gradually from there.

Patient sovereignty is not about perfection. It is about progress.

Every small step toward greater agency, better information, clearer communication, and more informed decision-making is a victory.

When the System Resists

I need to be honest: not all healthcare providers will welcome your newfound sovereignty. Some will feel threatened by patients who ask questions. Some will feel threatened by patients who bring data. Some will feel threatened by patients who insist on partnership. Some systems make it structurally difficult to practice what I am describing. They may offer secure messaging that you do not understand. They do not allow enough time for appointments. They do not support patient access to records.

When you encounter resistance, you have choices.

Educate. Sometimes providers resist because they do not understand what you are trying to do. Explaining that you are not questioning their expertise can shift the dynamic. You are trying to be a better partner. "I am bringing this data not because I do not trust you, but because I want to give you the most complete picture possible" can open doors.

Adapt. Sometimes you need to work within the system constraints. If your doctor will not engage with detailed symptom logs, maybe you distill them into a one-page summary. If secure messaging is not available, maybe you keep your own meticulous records. You can share them at appointments. Find workarounds that preserve your agency even in limiting systems.

Advocate. Sometimes the right response is to push for systemic change. Patient advocacy organizations are working to expand access to medical records. They are improving communication systems. They are supporting patient-centered care. Adding your voice to these efforts can create change that helps everyone.

Exit. Sometimes you need to find a different provider or system that better supports patient sovereignty. This is not always possible, but when it is, it can be transformative. Life is too short to stay in healthcare relationships that diminish rather than empower you.

The ultimate goal is not to force yourself to fit into a broken system. It is to practice sovereignty within whatever system you are in. Work toward better systems for everyone.

THE COMPOUNDING EFFECT

Here is what I have noticed after years of practicing these approaches systematically: the benefits compound.

The first time I prepared thoroughly for an appointment, it felt like a lot of work for modest improvement in that one visit. But that preparation created documentation I could reference for future visits. It established a pattern with my doctors of me showing up prepared and engaged. It built my confidence in advocating for myself. If nothing else it helped me consider my own healthcare more thoroughly.

The first time I tracked my symptoms carefully, I noticed some patterns but not dramatic insights. But months of data revealed trends that led to significant treatment improvements. The tracking became easier with practice. The AI-assisted analysis became more valuable as I accumulated more data.

The first time I used a decision-making framework for a medical choice, it felt academic and maybe overthought. But now, after using these frameworks repeatedly, they have become intuitive. I can quickly identify my values. I can assess evidence quality. I can evaluate reversibility almost automatically.

Each practice reinforces the others. Better documentation enables better preparation. Better tracking enables better communication. Better communication enables better decisions. Better decisions lead to better outcomes. Better outcomes reinforce your commitment to the practices.

This is the compounding effect of patient sovereignty. Small investments in agency accumulate into transformative change. In how you experience healthcare and how healthcare serves you.

You do not need to be perfect at any of this. You just need to be persistent. Keep practicing. Keep learning. Keep claiming your right to be a partner in your own care. The transformation happens not in dramatic moments. It happens in the steady accumulation of small acts of sovereignty.

This compounding effect extends beyond your own care. When you practice patient sovereignty consistently, you change the expectations of your healthcare providers. I have heard from doctors that working with engaged, prepared patients has made them better physicians. It has made them better physicians for all their patients, not just the prepared ones. They start routinely asking all their patients about what matters most. They invite patients to set agendas. They think out loud about trade-offs.

This is how systems change. Not through top-down mandates. But through bottom-up practice. Every patient who shows up prepared. Every patient who insists on partnership. Every patient who claims their right to understand and decide. These patients shift the culture of medicine a little bit. Those small shifts accumulate into transformation.

Your patient action plan is your declaration of sovereignty. It is a systematic approach to claiming your rightful place. You are the primary decision-maker in your healthcare. It is not about being perfect. It is not about having everything figured out. It is about having tools and frameworks. These support you in being as informed, prepared, and empowered as you can be. You do this at each stage of your journey.

Start small, build gradually, and trust that every step you take toward systematic engagement with your healthcare makes you more capable of the next step.

In the next chapter, we will zoom out from these individual practices. We will imagine what healthcare could look like if patient sovereignty became the norm rather than the exception. What becomes possible when patients are truly seen as sovereigns? What would the healthcare system need to look like to serve sovereign patients well? How do we get there from here?

Let us explore the healthcare you deserve.

Technology Note

The specific AI tools mentioned in this book (ChatGPT, Claude, Gemini) are examples of common tools and my suggestion is to use several of these tools. Compare results between tools and also share with them what you learned from another tool and watch how they respond. The principles in this chapter apply to any "Large Language Model" (LLM) AI tool. This applies regardless of the brand name. By the time you read this, new tools may have emerged. Current ones may have changed. Focus on the type of tool. Focus on conversational AI, symptom tracker, and medical research assistant. Do not focus on the specific company.

The sovereignty principles are what matters. The technology evolves, but the truths shared remain the same. Also, I am only speaking as a patient in my unique situation and what has worked for me. Both of our lived experiences are unique. Everyone is different. You need to find what works best for you. And throughout this process, work in concert with your healthcare provider.

13

THE HEALTHCARE YOU DESERVE

You have spent twelve chapters learning to claim your power inside a system that was not built for you. You know how to prepare for appointments, track your health data, ask the questions that matter, make decisions aligned with your values, and use AI as a tool for understanding. Those skills are real. They work. They can transform your experience with healthcare starting tomorrow.

This chapter is about something different. Not how to survive the system we have, but what the system could actually become. This is not a wish list. Real places in the real world are already building pieces of what you are about to read. The reason this matters to you personally: knowing what better healthcare looks like changes what you are willing to accept, what you demand, and what you help build.

Close Your Eyes for a Moment

Imagine walking into a clinic where the first question is not "What brings you in today?" but "What matters to you right now?" Imagine an appointment where there is enough time to actually answer that question honestly. Where your provider thinks out loud with you about diagnosis, explains the trade-offs between options, and asks what fits your life before writing a prescription.

Imagine your health record belongs to you. Every test result arrives in language you understand, not jargon. You can see exactly who accessed your data and when. When you move to a new city or see a new specialist, your information follows you seamlessly. No faxes. No duplicate tests. No starting over.

Imagine your doctor was trained from the first day of medical school to see you as a partner, not a problem to solve. Imagine their income did not depend on how many patients they could cycle through per hour, but on how well you were actually doing six months later. Imagine AI working quietly in the background, catching medication errors before they reach the pharmacy, flagging patterns in your data you might want to discuss, translating your radiology report into plain English the moment it posts.

None of this is science fiction. Every element I just described exists somewhere in the world right now. The pieces are scattered, fragmented, unevenly distributed. The question is not whether this kind of healthcare is possible. The question is whether we will connect the pieces.

It Is Already Happening

Estonia, a country of 1.3 million people, gives every citizen complete digital access to their health records. You can see who looked at your file, when they looked, and why. You control which providers see which information. The system is not perfect, but it proves something important: patient-controlled health information works at national scale. If a small country can do it, the infrastructure is not the barrier. The will is.

In the United States, direct primary care practices are offering something patients thought had disappeared forever: time. These practices run on membership models, not per-visit billing. A monthly fee covers your care. Appointments run forty-five to sixty minutes. Your doctor knows your name, your family, your fears. They are not trapped in the volume game that forces most physicians to see twenty-five patients a day in fifteen-minute windows. Concierge medicine has offered this to wealthy patients for years. Direct primary care is working to make it affordable for everyone.

Medical schools are beginning to teach partnership. Programs are emerging that focus on patient stories, shared decision-making, and motivational interviewing. Students are learning to ask "What matters to you?" as naturally as they ask "Where does it hurt?" These programs are still rare, and they compete for space in packed curricula. Making partnership central to being a good doctor requires more than adding a class. It requires rethinking what a good doctor is.

Payment models are shifting too, slowly. Accountable care organizations, patient-centered medical homes, and bundled payment models all create space for different kinds of provider-patient relationships. Instead of rewarding volume alone, these models begin to reward outcomes: how well you are doing, not just how many times you were seen. Early results are promising but not yet transformative. We need bolder experiments and faster adoption of what works.

Policy is moving in the right direction. The 21st Century Cures Act improved patient access to health data. Technical standards like FHIR are making it easier for different systems to share information. Regulations are slowly increasing your right to see your own records quickly and in usable formats. The pace is too slow. The scope is too limited. But the direction is clear.

What Is Still Standing in the Way

If all these pieces exist, why does your next doctor's appointment still feel the same? Because the system was not designed to take from you on purpose. It evolved that way, and the forces that shaped it are deeply entrenched.

Payment structures still reward speed over partnership. Providers get paid for visits, procedures, and tests, not for time spent understanding what matters to you. In this model, genuine collaboration is an economic loss. Technology was built for billing and legal protection, not to help you and your provider think together. Patient portals feel clunky because they were bolted on after the fact, never designed with you at the center. And the power imbalance is reinforced by everything from medical training to the physical layout of the exam room: the paper gown, the table, the doctor standing while the patient sits.

None of these barriers are permanent. Every one of them was built by human decisions, and human decisions can rebuild them. But it will not happen by accident. It requires people pushing from every direction at once.

Everyone Has a Role

System change does not happen all at once. It happens when enough people push from different positions at the same time. Bottom-up practice. Top-down policy. Small experiments proving what is possible. Successful models getting scaled up. Here is what each group can do right now.

What You Can Do

Every time you walk into an appointment prepared, with your questions organized and your data tracked, you show providers that patients can be genuine partners. Every time you ask for shared decision-making, you signal that the old pattern is not acceptable. Every time you choose a provider who collaborates with you, you create economic pressure for change. Your practice of sovereignty, multiplied across millions of patients, shifts expectations. Providers who work with engaged, prepared patients learn to value that engagement for all their patients, not just the prepared ones.

What Providers Can Do

Healthcare professionals who want to work in partnership with patients can start now, even within systems not designed for it. Think out loud about your diagnostic reasoning. Present options and trade-offs instead of directives. Acknowledge uncertainty. Respect patient time and agency. Within your organizations, push for longer appointments for complex cases, better communication tools, training in shared decision-making, and team-based care models that provide support between physician visits. And use the political power of professional organizations to advocate for payment reform, training reform, and technology reform.

What Policy Makers Can Do

Policy change is what makes patient power accessible to everyone, not just those with the resources to demand it. We need regulations that ensure patient access to health information, require systems to share data, and stop information blocking. We need payment reforms that recognize the value of time and partnership. We need funding for research on patient-centered care models and mechanisms to rapidly scale what works. We need medical education reform that makes partnership core to professional training.

What Technology Companies Can Do

Technology companies entering healthcare need to center patient power in their design choices instead of optimizing for efficiency or profit alone. Build AI tools that support decision-making without replacing human relationships. Create health information systems that patients actually control. Make algorithms transparent and explainable. Companies that do this will build what patients actually want once patients have the power to choose. Getting there means resisting short-term incentives that optimize system efficiency at the expense of patient autonomy.

Technology as Partner, Not Master

If there is one thing I have learned about technology and patient power, it is this: technology is essential, but it is not enough. And it can do real harm if it is deployed without centering human relationship.

AI can help you analyze your health data, identify patterns, translate complex medical information into language you understand, prepare for appointments, track your progress between visits, catch errors, and flag concerning trends. It can reduce the knowledge gap that creates the power difference in healthcare. You have already seen this throughout the earlier chapters.

But AI can also deepen extraction if we are not careful. An AI that replaces conversation with your doctor makes things worse, not better. A system that uses your data to optimize provider efficiency instead of your outcomes serves the wrong master. Technology designed to monitor your compliance and push you into following rules undermines your sovereignty instead of strengthening it.

The difference comes down to one question: was this technology built to serve your power, or to optimize the system? Those goals sometimes overlap. Often they do not. A healthcare system designed around you would answer that question the same way every time: your power comes first.

What Becomes Possible

When healthcare is redesigned around patient power, things that seem utopian now become entirely achievable with existing knowledge and technology.

Medical errors decrease because patients are empowered to catch them. Treatment adherence improves because plans are designed collaboratively around what is actually feasible in your life. Health disparities narrow because partnership surfaces the life circumstances that drive poor health. Trust in healthcare improves because you experience the system as genuinely working for you, not extracting from you.

Innovation accelerates because you become a source of insight, not just a research subject. Chronic disease management improves because you have the tools and support to be an effective partner in your own care. Prevention becomes more effective because it is designed around what you actually value, not what experts think you should value.

Healthcare becomes more human. You feel seen as a whole person, not a collection of symptoms and billing codes. Providers find more meaning in their work because they are building genuine relationships instead of processing cases. The anxiety and disconnection that characterize so much of healthcare begin to diminish.

These outcomes are already being achieved in pockets, in healthcare systems and practices that have committed to patient-centered partnership. The question is not whether this is possible. The question is whether we have the will to make it universal.

The Healthcare You Deserve

You deserve healthcare that sees you as a person with power, not a subject. You deserve providers who ask what matters to you, not just what is wrong with you. You deserve time for real conversation. You deserve complete access to your own health information in language you can understand. You deserve partnership in decisions that affect your body and your life.

You deserve healthcare that adapts to your actual life instead of demanding you adapt to ideal protocols. You deserve technology that serves your needs instead of monitoring your compliance. You deserve care that helps you live according to your values, not someone else's definition of optimal health.

This is not asking for too much. In a society that claims to value human dignity and autonomy, this is the bare minimum.

The gap between the healthcare system we have and the system you deserve is wide, but it is not unbridgeable. The tools exist. The knowledge exists. Examples of healthcare delivered differently exist. What is required is the collective will to demand something better and the sustained effort to build it.

Your practice of sovereignty, the tools and frameworks throughout this book, is part of that building. Every prepared appointment. Every partnership conversation. Every informed decision. Every insistence on being treated as a whole person with agency. These shift the culture of healthcare, one encounter at a time. Those shifts accumulate. They change provider expectations. They create demand for different models of care. They make the next shift easier.

The healthcare system will not transform overnight. But it is transforming. You can be part of that transformation by claiming your power within the system that exists and demanding the system that should exist.

The coming chapters will bring us full circle, back to where you are right now: living with a health condition, navigating an imperfect system, trying to be well. We will talk about what it means to practice sovereignty day by day, how to sustain it over time, and why it matters beyond your individual experience.

Take a moment with the vision in this chapter. Let yourself feel what it would be like to experience healthcare that truly serves you. Let yourself believe it is possible. Because it is. And believing it is possible is the first step toward making it real.

14

———

PRACTICING SOVEREIGNTY IN REAL LIFE

COMING FULL CIRCLE

We're back where we started: you, living with a health condition, navigating an imperfect healthcare system, trying to be well. Working to understand the concepts of patient sovereignty over time, navigating the inevitable setbacks with grace, and finding meaning in the daily practice of being as well as possible.

Reading this book hasn't cured your condition. It hasn't transformed the healthcare system. You still have appointments that feel rushed. You still have doctors who don't quite get it. You still have days when your symptoms are overwhelming and the last thing you want to think about is being a "sovereign patient."

But something has shifted.

You now have language for what was wrong with those transactional appointments. You have tools for organizing your health information and preparing for visits. You have frameworks for making decisions that align with what actually matters to you. You have permission to ask for what you need, to ask to be heard, to take your place as a partner in your own care.

The question isn't whether you know what to do. The question is: How do you keep doing it? Not just this week or this month, but over the months and years of living with a chronic condition? How do you sustain this practice when you're tired, when you're discouraged, when you've had three bad appointments in a row and you're wondering if any of this actually makes a difference?

That's what this chapter is about. Not the theory of patient sovereignty or the vision of what healthcare could be. The messy, daily, imperfect reality of trying to practice sovereignty over time.

Because here's what I've learned after years of this: Sovereignty isn't a destination you reach. It's a practice you maintain. And maintaining any practice over time (especially when you're managing a chronic condition) requires something different than just knowing what to do. It requires compassion for yourself, realistic expectations, strategies for hard times, and a deep understanding of why the practice matters even when individual moments feel futile.

This is the chapter about the long game.

The Reality of Living Sovereign

Let me tell you what practicing sovereignty actually looks like in real life.

Some days, you'll prepare for an appointment beautifully. You'll have your questions written down, your symptoms tracked, and your priorities clear. The appointment will go well. You'll feel heard. You'll leave with a plan that makes sense. You'll think, "Yes, this sovereignty thing works."

Other days, you'll be too exhausted to prepare. You'll drag yourself to the appointment, barely holding it together. You'll forget half of what you meant to say. The doctor will be rushed or dismissive. You'll leave feeling defeated and wondering why you even tried.

Some weeks, you'll track your symptoms consistently, notice helpful patterns, and feel like you're gaining insight into your condition. Other weeks, you'll be too sick or too overwhelmed to track anything, and you'll beat yourself up about it.

Some medical encounters will confirm everything you've learned in this book about partnership and collaboration. Others will make you want to scream because you're right back in the extraction paradigm (the system that treats healthcare like a transaction: extract information, extract compliance, extract payment, without regard for your life context or what matters to you).

And here's the hardest part: practicing sovereignty doesn't guarantee good health outcomes. You can do everything "right" (prepare perfectly, communicate clearly, advocate effectively) and still have your symptoms worsen. You can be the most engaged, informed, sovereign patient in the world, and still experience the frustration of treatments that don't work, diagnoses that take too long, and a healthcare system that fails you in moments when you need it most.

This is the reality that no book on patient empowerment wants to address. But I'm going to talk about it because pretending otherwise sets you up for failure and self-blame.

Sovereignty doesn't cure your condition. It doesn't fix the systemic problems in healthcare. What it does (what it's supposed to do) is give you more agency in navigating an imperfect system while managing an imperfect body. That's it. That's all it can do.

And some days, that will feel like enough. Other days, it will feel like trying to bail water out of a sinking ship with a teaspoon.

Both of those experiences are part of practicing sovereignty over time. The good days don't mean you're "doing it right," and the bad days don't mean you're failing. They're both just part of the reality of living with a chronic condition in a healthcare system that wasn't designed for your needs.

The practice isn't about eliminating the bad days. It's about showing up consistently (even imperfectly) and maintaining your sense of agency even when outcomes aren't what you hoped.

Practice, Not Perfection

Here's something I wish I'd understood earlier: The goal isn't to be perfect at patient sovereignty. The goal is to keep practicing.

Think about any other long-term practice: meditation, exercise, learning an instrument. Nobody expects perfection. You don't meditate perfectly every day. You don't have a perfect workout every time. You don't play every piece of music flawlessly. The practice is about showing up consistently, doing what you can with the capacity you have that day, and trusting that the cumulative effect matters more than any individual session.

Patient sovereignty works the same way.

You won't prepare perfectly for every appointment. Some days, "preparation" will be scribbling three questions on a Post-it note in the waiting room. That's okay. That's still practice.

You won't communicate perfectly in every medical encounter. Some days, you'll forget to ask important questions or fail to speak up when you should. That's okay. That's part of learning.

You won't make optimal decisions every time. Some choices will turn out badly. Some paths you take will dead-end. That's okay. That's part of the process.

The perfection trap is especially seductive for people managing chronic conditions. We so desperately want to gain control over something in our lives that we can become rigid about the practices that are supposed to help us. We turn "prepare for appointments" into an all-or-nothing mandate where anything less than perfect preparation feels like failure. We turn "track your symptoms" into a source of anxiety where missing a day of tracking triggers shame and self-criticism.

This is the opposite of sovereignty. Sovereignty includes the freedom to practice imperfectly, to have bad days, to adjust your approach based on your current capacity, and to be human.

This perfection trap is real and surprisingly common. Some patients become so rigorous about symptom tracking that the tracking itself becomes a source of anxiety and misery. Tracking everything (sleep, food, stress, symptoms, medications) multiple times a day. Thinking this makes them a "good" sovereign patient when actually, the practice is making them sicker than the condition itself.

The practice of sovereignty should make your life better, not add another source of stress. If your approach to practicing sovereignty is making you more anxious, more perfectionistic, or more miserable, something's wrong. You've confused rigorous practice with effective practice. You've made sovereignty itself into a tyranny.

When this happens, the solution is to scale back. Track only what matters most for your specific medical decisions. Give yourself permission to track nothing on some days. Your healthcare won't fall apart. You can still be an effective partner to your doctors. You just do it with more self-compassion and less self-imposed pressure.

Because here's the truth: A sustainable imperfect practice beats an unsustainable perfect practice every time.

MINIMAL VIABLE SOVEREIGNTY ON BAD DAYS

When you're at your lowest capacity, sovereignty can look like:

- Show up to the appointment (even unprepared is better than missing it)
- Bring one trusted person who knows what matters to you
- Have your one-page medical summary accessible (diagnoses, meds, allergies)

When You're Too Tired to Advocate

There will be times when you're too sick, too exhausted, or too depleted to advocate for yourself. This is especially true if you're managing a chronic condition that affects your energy, cognition, or emotional capacity.

During my worst seizure clusters, I can barely string sentences together, let alone prepare for appointments or advocate effectively in medical conversations. During those times, the idea of practicing patient sovereignty feels laughable. I'm just trying to survive the day.

If you're living with a chronic condition, you know this experience. The times when your condition flares so badly that all your energy goes to basic functioning. The periods of treatment side effects that leave you too foggy or exhausted to do anything beyond what's absolutely necessary. The emotional lows where even answering your doctor's questions feels overwhelming.

During these times, the practice of sovereignty looks different. It's not about optimal engagement. It's about minimal viable sovereignty: whatever version of agency you can maintain with the capacity you currently have.

This is where planning during your high-capacity periods pays off. During the times when you're feeling relatively well and thinking clearly, you can set up systems that help you during low-capacity periods:

Keep a one-page summary of your essential health information (diagnoses, current medications, allergies, emergency contacts) that you or someone else can grab quickly when needed.

Identify one or two people who can advocate for you when you can't advocate for yourself. Talk to them ahead of time about what matters to you, what questions they should ask, what decisions you'd want to make in various scenarios.

Set up communication with your healthcare team that doesn't require real-time conversation. Patient portal messaging, email, text updates: whatever allows you to share important information when you have capacity rather than requiring immediate response.

Create decision frameworks during well times so you have guidelines during crisis times. "If X happens, I want to try Y before Z." You can't make complex decisions when you're depleted, but you can follow frameworks you created when you were clear-headed.

Lower your definition of "successful" practice during hard times. Maybe preparation means just showing up to the appointment. Maybe advocacy means having someone else speak for you. Maybe tracking means writing one sentence a day. That's enough. That's still practice.

And here's the permission you might need: It's okay to have seasons where you're barely practicing sovereignty at all. Where you're just getting through. Where healthcare is happening to you more than you're actively shaping it. Sometimes survival is the practice. Sometimes just making it through is enough.

The goal isn't to maintain peak sovereignty all the time. The goal is to do what you can with what you have, and to be compassionate with yourself about what you can't do.

After Setbacks: Getting Back On the Horse

You will have setbacks. Guaranteed.

You'll have an appointment that goes terribly despite your best preparation. You'll have a health crisis that knocks you completely off your sovereignty practice. You'll have periods where you fall out of all your good habits (no tracking, no preparation, no advocacy) because you're just too overwhelmed or too discouraged.

The skill you need isn't how to avoid setbacks. It's how to restart after them.

I've had to restart my sovereignty practice more times than I can count. Sometimes because my health deteriorated and I couldn't maintain the practice. Sometimes because I got discouraged after a series of bad medical encounters and stopped trying. Sometimes because life got overwhelming and healthcare fell to the bottom of my priority list. Sometimes for no clear reason at all: I just drifted away from the practice and woke up one day realizing I hadn't prepared for an appointment or tracked a symptom in months.

Every time, I had to figure out how to begin again.

Restarting After You Begin to Drift

When you notice you've drifted from your practice:

1. **Focus on the small wins.** For me, if I do just one small thing to practice my sovereignty, I've won. This could be something as simple as going for a walk outside, doing one simple stretch, calling a friend, going shopping, or, if I'm really struggling, this might mean just showering (if

you face a really hard day you know what I'm talking about), doing just one part of my morning routine. Sometimes just showing up in life is enough.

2. Pick ONE simple practice to restart (just write three questions before your next appointment).

3. Reconnect with why it matters to you personally (not because you "should").

4. Set a specific restart trigger ("Sunday 3 pm: review health dashboard for Tuesday appointment").

5. Remember, our journey is a marathon, not a sprint.

Here's what I've learned about restarting:

Start small. When you're getting back to practice after a break, the temptation is to do everything at once to "make up for" the time you weren't practicing. This almost always fails. Instead, pick one practice (just one) and restart with that. Maybe it's just writing down three questions before your next appointment. Maybe it's tracking one symptom. Maybe it's sending one update message to your doctor. Start there. Build back gradually.

Resist the shame spiral. Your brain will want to tell you that you failed, that you're bad at this, that you should have maintained the practice all along. Don't indulge that voice. You didn't fail. You're human. You had other priorities or less capacity or harder circumstances. None of that means the practice doesn't work or that you're not capable of doing it. It just means you took a break. Now you're starting again. That's how practices work.

Reconnect with why it matters. Before you jump back into the how of sovereignty practice, remind yourself of the why. Why does this matter to you? What difference did it make when you were practicing consistently? What do you want from your healthcare that sovereignty helps you achieve? Reconnecting with purpose makes the restart feel meaningful rather than obligatory.

Adjust your approach. If you drifted away from your practice, ask yourself if the way you were doing it was actually sustainable. Maybe you need a simpler version. Maybe you need different tools.

Maybe you need to lower the bar for what counts as "success." Use the restart as an opportunity to refine your practice, not just resume the version that wasn't working.

Set a specific restart trigger. As I shared previously, this might mean "I'll start preparing for appointments again" is vague. "I'll spend 20 minutes on Sunday afternoon reviewing my health dashboard and writing questions for my Tuesday appointment" is specific. Give yourself a clear action plan and timeline for restarting.

The pattern you want to build is this: Practice → Drift → Notice → Restart → Practice. **Not:** Practice → Drift → Shame → Give up.

The practice of sovereignty isn't a straight line. It's a cycle. And the more comfortable you get with the restart part of the cycle, the less the drift part will feel like failure.

The Cumulative Effect You Won't See Coming

Here's what surprised me about practicing sovereignty over years rather than weeks: The benefits compound in ways you won't predict.

In the short term (the first few appointments where you practice preparation and advocacy) you might notice modest improvements. Maybe one question gets answered that wouldn't have been. Maybe you feel slightly more heard. Maybe you catch one small error. These improvements matter, but they can feel incremental. You might wonder if all this effort is worth it.

But over months and years, something shifts that you won't see coming.

Your relationship with your healthcare providers changes. Doctors who work with you consistently start to expect your engagement. They adjust how they communicate. They think out loud with you because they've learned you want to be part of the reasoning process. They ask what matters to you because they've learned that's important to the conversation. The partnership you've been practicing starts to feel less like something you work toward and more like the default mode of your relationship.

Your relationship with your condition changes. You move from feeling like a victim of your illness to feeling like someone managing a challenging situation. Your condition doesn't improve (mine certainly hasn't), but your sense of agency does. You stop waiting for your healthcare team to fix you and start seeing yourself as the primary manager of your wellbeing, with your healthcare team as expert consultants. This shift in identity matters more than any specific health outcome.

Your capacity for advocacy grows without you noticing. Things that felt hard and scary early in your practice (asking clarifying questions, disagreeing with a recommendation, requesting more time) become easier. Not because the system gets less intimidating, but because you've practiced these skills enough that they feel more natural. You develop confidence in your ability to navigate medical conversations that you didn't have before.

Your health literacy deepens. After years of asking questions, researching your condition, tracking patterns, and making decisions, you develop a level of expertise about your own health that becomes genuinely valuable. You can spot concerning symptoms early. You can identify patterns your doctors miss. You can evaluate treatment options with nuance. This knowledge compounds over time.

The Weekly 10-Minute Reset

Set a weekly time to:

- Review your symptom patterns from the past week
- Note one question or concern for your next visit
- Update your one-page medical summary if anything changed

These cumulative effects take time. You won't see them after a month or even six months. But after a year or two of consistent practice, you'll look back and realize something fundamental has changed. Not your health status necessarily, but your capacity to navigate health challenges with agency and resilience.

That's the long game. That's what you're building toward.

Why Your Practice Matters Beyond You

Some days, when you're exhausted and discouraged, you might wonder: Why keep doing this? I'm just one person. What difference does it really make?

I want to tell you why it matters. Not just for you, but beyond you.

Every time you show up to an appointment prepared, you're teaching your healthcare providers what engaged partnership looks like. Many doctors trained in an era where patient passivity was expected. When they encounter patients who are informed, organized, and ready to collaborate, it can challenge their assumptions. It shows them a different way of practicing medicine is possible. Some resist. But many don't. Many recognize that working with engaged patients is often more satisfying and can lead to better outcomes.

Every time you ask to be heard, to have your questions answered, to be part of decisions about your body, you're creating space for patients who come after you. The patients who don't have your resources, your education, your confidence, or your capacity to advocate. When you raise the bar for what patients expect, it can make the system more responsive to everyone.

For those of us who have access and leverage (whether that's time to prepare, transportation to appointments, a support person who can come with us, or comfort navigating patient portals), using those advantages to advocate for better care isn't just personal. It can create conditions that benefit others. When a doctor learns to listen to engaged patients, they may become more attuned to all their patients. When a clinic adjusts its processes because patients speak up, everyone benefits.

Every time you share your sovereignty practices with friends, family, or patient communities, you're spreading tools and permission. You're modeling what's possible. You're helping others learn what you learned the hard way. The practices you share might help someone navigate a diagnosis you've never faced, in circumstances you've never experienced.

Your practice is part of something larger than your individual healthcare journey. Whether you intended it or not, whether you ever see the effects or not, your consistent practice of sovereignty can contribute to a slow cultural shift in how healthcare works.

This doesn't mean you're responsible for fixing the system. You're not. The burden of transformation rests with institutions, policymakers, and healthcare leaders, not with individual patients who are already managing chronic conditions. But it does mean your practice has meaning beyond its immediate utility to you.

On the hard days, when you're questioning whether any of this makes a difference, remember: You're advocating for yourself and your own wellbeing. That's the primary goal. That's enough. And sometimes, as a side effect, your practice helps create conditions for better care for others too.

What Success Actually Looks Like

Let me tell you what success doesn't look like in sovereignty practice:

- It doesn't look like perfect health. For many of us the condition and/or symptoms won't disappear because you practiced sovereignty well.
- It doesn't look like zero frustration with the healthcare system. You'll still encounter barriers, inefficiencies, and failures.
- It doesn't look like never having bad appointments. Even the best-prepared patient will sometimes work with providers who can't or won't practice partnership.
- It doesn't look like always feeling confident and capable. You'll still have moments of doubt, fear, and feeling overwhelmed.

If those are your metrics for success, you'll always feel like you're failing. Because those aren't realistic outcomes of sovereignty practice. They're fantasies about what healthcare or chronic illness management could be if the world were fundamentally different from what it is.

So what does success actually look like?

Success is showing up consistently, even when it's hard. It's preparing for appointments more often than not. It's asking at least some of your important questions most of the time. It's tracking symptoms when you have capacity. It's advocating for yourself even when it feels awkward. Consistency, not perfection, is the metric.

Success is learning from your experiences. It's noticing when something works and doing more of it. It's recognizing when an approach isn't serving you and adjusting it. It's getting slightly better at preparation, communication, or decision-making over time. Growth, not mastery, is the metric.

Success is maintaining agency even in difficult moments. It's feeling like a partner in your care even when outcomes aren't what you hoped. It's making informed decisions even when all your options are imperfect. It's believing your voice matters even when you're not sure you're being heard. Agency, not control, is the metric.

Success is celebrating small wins. Caught one error. Asked one good question. Felt heard in one conversation. Left one appointment with clarity instead of confusion. These matter. These accumulate. These are success.

Success is being kinder to yourself about the hard parts. It's having self-compassion when you're too tired to advocate. It's restarting without shame after you've drifted from your practice. It's accepting your limits without seeing them as failures. Compassion, not self-criticism, is the metric.

Success is tracking your progress over months, not days. It's looking back three months or six months or a year and noticing that something has shifted: your confidence, your relationship with your providers, your capacity to navigate hard situations. Long-term trajectory, not daily perfection, is the metric.

If you can do most of these things most of the time (even imperfectly), you're succeeding at sovereignty practice. Even when it doesn't feel like success. Even when you're still frustrated with the system or struggling with your health. Even when you look around and feel like everyone else is doing it better.

Success in sovereignty practice looks like showing up as the fullest version of yourself that you can be on that particular day, with that particular capacity, in that particular situation. That's it. That's enough.

The Permission to Be Human

You need to give yourself permission for something, in case you need to hear it:

You don't have to be perfect at patient sovereignty. You don't even have to be good at it all the time. You're allowed to be human.

You're allowed to have appointments where you forget every question you meant to ask. Where you nod along even though you're confused. Where you say "yes" to something you're not sure about because you're too overwhelmed to advocate for yourself in that moment. That doesn't make you a bad patient or a failed sovereign. It makes you human.

You're allowed to be angry at the healthcare system. To rage against the unfairness of having a chronic condition. To feel bitter about the time and energy you have to spend managing your health instead of living your life. Those feelings are valid. They don't contradict sovereignty. They're part of the emotional reality of living with illness in a broken system.

You're allowed to take breaks from active advocacy. To have periods where you're just coasting, just getting through, just doing the bare minimum. You don't have to be optimally engaged with your healthcare all the time. Sometimes survival is the only goal, and that's legitimate.

You're allowed to prioritize other parts of your life over healthcare management. Your health is important, but it's not the only important thing. Sometimes your relationships, your work, your creative pursuits, or your mental health need to take precedence. You're allowed to choose that.

You're allowed to just be tired. Tired of appointments. Tired of medications. Tired of tracking symptoms. Tired of explaining your condition to new providers. Tired of the constant cognitive and emotional labor of managing a chronic illness. That exhaustion is real and valid. You don't have to perform enthusiasm for sovereignty practice when you're just worn out.

You're allowed to need help. To ask for support. To let other people advocate for you when you can't do it yourself. Sovereignty doesn't mean doing everything alone. It means having agency over your care, which sometimes includes the agency to delegate, to ask for help, to lean on others.

You're allowed to have bad days, bad weeks, bad months. Where the practice falls apart. Where you're barely holding on. Where sovereignty feels like a luxury you can't afford because you're too busy just trying to survive. Those times don't erase the value of the practice or mean you've failed. They're just part of the reality of living with a chronic condition.

I'm saying all this because books about patient empowerment can accidentally create a new form of pressure. You read about all these tools and frameworks and practices, and suddenly you feel like you should be doing all of it perfectly all the time. Like if you're not optimally sovereign, you're failing.

That's not what this book is for. This book is meant to give you options, not obligations. Tools, not requirements. Permission, not pressure.

Use what helps. Let go of what doesn't. Adjust everything to fit your actual life, your actual capacity, your actual circumstances. Practice sovereignty in whatever form works for you, even if it looks nothing like what's described in these chapters.

Because here's the truth: The goal isn't to turn you into the perfect sovereign patient. The goal is to help you be more fully yourself in your healthcare journey. And being fully yourself includes being imperfect, being tired, being human.

You're allowed. All of it. You're allowed.

The Journey Continues

We've reached a turning point in this book, but not the end of your journey. Tomorrow you'll wake up still living with your condition. You'll still need to navigate the healthcare system. You'll still have appointments and decisions and moments when you're not sure what to do.

But you're better equipped now than when you started.

You understand why healthcare often feels so transactional and what you can do about it. You know how AI is already shaping your care and how to use it as a tool for your sovereignty. You have frameworks for organizing your health information, preparing for appointments, and making decisions that align with what matters to you. You know how to ask better questions, build your healthcare team, and have transformative conversations with providers.

None of this guarantees easy answers or good outcomes. But it gives you agency. It gives you tools. It gives you permission to be a partner in your own care.

The practice continues tomorrow, and the day after that. Some days will go well. Many days will be harder than you'd like. All of it is part of the practice.

I won't lie to you and say it gets easy. Managing a chronic condition never gets easy. Navigating a broken healthcare system never gets easy. But it can get more bearable. It can feel less like something happening to you and more like something you're actively navigating.

I'm 61 years old, living with a traumatic brain injury and epilepsy that will never be cured. I've been practicing sovereignty imperfectly for years now. I still have bad days. I still have appointments that frustrate me. I still struggle with symptoms that derail my plans and complicate my life.

But I'm not the same person I was when I started this journey. I've learned to define what matters to me and to make decisions aligned with those values. I've learned to communicate effectively with my healthcare team and to be a genuine partner in my care. I've learned to use tools (including AI) to support my agency rather than replace it. I've learned to practice sovereignty imperfectly and to be compassionate with myself when I fall short.

Most importantly, I've learned that I deserve to be seen as fully human in my pursuit of wellness. Not just as a patient with a condition, but as a person with a life.

You deserve that too. You deserve healthcare that sees you, hears you, and partners with you. You deserve providers who ask what matters to you, not just what's wrong with you.

The tools are in this book. The permission is yours. The practice is available whenever you're ready.

You've already started just by reading this far. That's enough for today.

15

WHAT'S COMING: THE FUTURE OF AI IN YOUR CARE

You've built your toolkit. You know how to prepare for appointments, ask better questions, and partner with your care team. Now I want to show you what's coming next — because AI in healthcare isn't slowing down, and what you've learned so far will matter even more in the months and years ahead.

Some of what I describe in this chapter is already available. Some is being tested in clinics and research labs. Some is still years out. I'll mark each section so you know where things stand. But here's what I want you to hold onto: the skills you've been practicing throughout this book — staying informed, asking questions, insisting on partnership — are exactly what you'll need as these technologies arrive.

A few ideas will come up repeatedly. Treatments designed for your specific body, not for the average patient. Computer systems making recommendations about your care. Your right to have a real person review those recommendations when an AI says "no." These are the themes running through everything ahead, and I'll explain each one as we get there.

Let's start with how fast this is moving.

The Acceleration Is Here

Most people miss something important about AI. It doesn't improve slowly. It accelerates fast. Very fast.

Think about electricity. Think about the internet. Think about smartphones. Each took decades to become normal. Slow adoption. Slow building. Gradual change. AI is different. Change is fast. It's exciting and unsettling.

Consider this fact. In 2023, about 38% of U.S. doctors used AI. By 2024, that jumped to 66%. Nearly doubled in one year and those numbers have grown exponentially ever since.

This adoption rate shows fast growth. But more tools doesn't automatically mean better patient care. The global AI healthcare market was worth about 39 billion dollars in 2025. Experts say it will reach 500 billion by 2032. This shows industry confidence. But researchers are still checking which AI actually helps patients.

I started thinking seriously about AI healthcare several years ago. I realized AI tools were improving faster than I could learn about them. Some AI tools I read about in research papers seemed far away. Things maybe five or ten years away. Now, as I write, those tools are already being tested. By the time you read this, even more will be available. Change is happening fast.

This speed matters for your healthcare in good ways and concerning ways. AI systems work behind the scenes in your care right now. You read about these in earlier chapters. Soon you'll see them more. They'll do more things. They'll touch every part of your healthcare.

Some changes will truly help you control your health better. AI tools will give you new information. They'll give you support you never had before. They'll help you understand your condition more deeply. You'll prepare better for appointments. You'll make decisions with more confidence.

But some changes threaten your control if we're not careful. AI systems without good supervision threaten your autonomy. AI systems without your input threaten your power. AI systems that ignore fairness and consent can turn you into a data point. They stop treating you as a partner in your care.

The future isn't fixed. Technology companies and healthcare systems will make certain choices. But you matter too. Patients like you can influence this. You need to make sure AI serves your needs. AI shouldn't replace human doctors.

This chapter prepares you for what's coming. Not with fear, but with knowledge. Not by fighting all change, but with clear ways to judge which changes help you stay in control. Which changes harm your control.

Change is happening, and you can be ready for it.

TIMELINE: WHAT'S AVAILABLE WHEN

THROUGHOUT THIS CHAPTER, YOU'LL SEE THESE LABELS:

[AVAILABLE TODAY] = In use now at many healthcare systems
    [NEAR HORIZON] = In testing; may be available in 1-3 years
    [EXPERIMENTAL] = Early research; 3-5+ years from common use

AI Companions for Emotional & Medical Support [NEAR HORIZON]

One huge change coming in healthcare AI is emotional support chatbots. These are built to specifically help people living with chronic illness.

Right now, between doctor visits, your emotional support options are limited. You can call a friend. You can post in an online community. You can journal. You can wait for therapy. And only if you can access mental health care.

Soon you'll have another choice. AI companions trained to support people with complex medical conditions.

These aren't simple customer service chatbots. Those give unhelpful generic answers. The new AI companions are much smarter. They can have detailed, caring conversations. They adapt to your specific needs. They respond to how you're feeling.

Imagine support at 3 AM when anxiety wakes you. Imagine talking through your fears about new treatment. Imagine not burdening loved ones. Imagine a conversation partner who knows your medical history. They understand how your condition affects you. They help you work through what you're struggling with.

This is coming. Parts are already being tested.

Researchers studied these tools closely. One of the most comprehensive reviews to date, published in 2025, examined 25 different studies. These studies examined AI agents that help people manage chronic diseases. A separate analysis of 30 studies found something equally important. They looked at how well AI companions communicate. The findings? When designed well, these tools help patients feel better about their care. They improve emotional well-being.

Real users already experience this in pilot programs. Researchers studied over 150 reviews. People using the Wysa mental health app were studied. This was between 2020 and 2024. Users consistently said the AI companion helped them feel connected. It encouraged positive steps. It supported their emotional strength. However, please note that current tools are not designed to address clinical needs; I'm referring to clinically graded tools, not simple chatbots.

CRITICAL SAFETY BOUNDARY:

AI companions help process emotions. They are not medical tools. They can't:

- Diagnose medical emergencies
- Stop a mental health crisis
- Replace a licensed therapist
- Replace emergency services

If you're experiencing a medical emergency, suicidal thoughts, or severe mental health crisis, call 911. Call the 988 Suicide & Crisis Lifeline. Go to your nearest emergency room. AI companions provide emotional support between doctor visits. They're not crisis help.

Let's be clear about what AI companions can and can't do outside emergencies. This matters.

Current AI companions can listen without judgment. They work 24 hours a day, 7 days a week. They help you organize your thoughts and feelings. They provide information and perspective. They help you prepare for tough conversations with your healthcare team. They witness your experience. They reflect back what you're expressing. This helps you process it.

But they can't replace real human connection.

They can't provide the support that comes from someone who knows you deeply. They don't know your complete history. They don't know your habits when you aren't in front of your computer. They don't understand your unspoken needs. They are tools, not relationships.

And here's an important limit. These AI companions show real promise. But they're still being rigorously tested. A 2024 review of mental health AI chatbots found something concerning. Of 160 studies examining these tools from 2020-2024, only 16% of the studies on newer systems included rigorous clinical testing. This means conversational AI is advancing faster than our ability to thoroughly test their clinical effectiveness.

The goal isn't for AI to replace your therapist. It's not to replace your support group. It's not to replace your best friend. The goal is to give you one more resource. One that's always available. Never exhausted by your needs. Specifically designed to support your emotional wellbeing between human support.

Used well, AI companions can potentially help you process emotions more effectively, but they can also exhibit something called "toxic positivity" which you can research more through your favorite AI tool. The current tools can support better decision-making processes and communication tips with your care provider. They become part of your control toolkit. Another way to maintain control over your emotional experience of illness.

Used poorly, as a complete replacement for human connection, they can cause isolation and severe harm. They can disconnect you from people and communities that support you. Real people who care about you. Also, I would never trust any of these current tools with medical advice, ever! In fact, most of them have guardrails to stop themselves from giving you medical advice.

As these tools become more available, ask yourself this. Does this AI help me show up fully in my human relationships? Does it help me show up fully in my healthcare partnerships? Or does it help me avoid those connections? The first serves your control. The second undermines it.

"TREATMENT MATCHED TO YOU" GETS REAL [AVAILABLE TODAY / EXPANDING - CLINICIANS ONLY]

You've probably heard about "treatment matched to you" for years. It's been promised for a while. The idea that treatments would fit your specific body. Your genetic makeup. Your individual response patterns.

AI is about to make this promise real.

Right now, most treatment plans work like this. You have Condition X. So you try Treatment Y because that's what works for most people with Condition X. If it doesn't work for you, you try Treatment Z. Then maybe Treatment A. It's educated guessing. It's based on statistics about groups. Those groups might not be like you at all.

This approach wastes months, sometimes years, of your life. You take treatments that were never going to work for your specific body.

AI changes this in basic ways. Instead of relying on group averages, AI can analyze huge datasets. It identifies patterns that predict who responds to which treatments. It looks at hundreds of variables at once. Your specific symptoms. Your genetics. Your lifestyle. Your past treatment responses. AI can process all of this together. It suggests treatments most likely to work for you.

The progress is striking. In 2024, the FDA approved 47 new drugs.

Eighteen of them, about 38%, were treatment-matched to you. They were designed for specific patient groups. Not everyone with a condition. That's a significant shift.

And innovation is speeding up. In March 2025, a drug called Rentosertib became the first medication designed by AI to get an official name from regulators. This is a major milestone. The timeline is striking. This drug went from initial discovery to human trials in under 30 months. Using traditional methods takes 5-10 years.

For you, this means fewer failed treatments. Fewer months on medications that don't work. Faster paths to treatments that actually help. More precision. Less guessing.

But, and this is crucial, AI recommendations are only as good as the information they learned from.

Here's the problem. If the datasets used to train AI systems don't include many people like you, the predictions may be less accurate. If you're a woman, a person of color, someone over 65, or someone in a rural area, you're at risk. These groups have historically been under-represented in medical research. AI treatment matching might work less well for you than for well-studied groups. Typically, those are white men in urban academic medical centers.

This is where your control practice matters. When your doctor presents an AI treatment recommendation, ask these questions that actually get useful answers.

CLINICAL AGENCY QUESTIONS YOU MUST ASK YOUR DOCTOR:

None of these tools should be done without first talking to your healthcare provider.

"In your experience, does this AI recommendation work for patients like me with my specific [lifestyle factor/ethnicity/age/other condition]?" Your doctor can actually answer this. They can answer based on their experience with similar patients. This is more useful than asking about "information used to teach the AI." Your doctor likely doesn't know those details.

"How confident are you that this will work for someone like me with my specific presentation? What factors create uncertainty?" This asks your doctor to use their clinical judgment. Not a technical error rate. Your doctor can discuss what makes them more or less certain. They can discuss this for your specific case.

"If this doesn't work for me, what's our backup plan?" This is the critical question. Your doctor's expertise shines here. They can walk you through next steps. They can discuss alternative approaches. They can explain how you'll know together if you need to change direction. This is collaborative medicine at its best.

"Are there alternative approaches we should consider based on my specific values and priorities?" The AI ranks options by likelihood of success. But you might have priorities that matter more. Side effects matter. Lifestyle impact matters. Cost matters. These might make a lower-ranked option better for your actual life.

"How will we monitor whether this is working, and when do we decide to try something else?" Clear success metrics and timeline agreements. This is a partnership, not just a prescription.

Notice what these questions do. They leverage your doctor's clinical judgment and experience. They focus on your individual case. Not abstract algorithmic details. They create a collaborative plan with clear next steps.

AI can make medicine more treatment matched to you. But you're still the most important variable in the equation. The technology should inform decisions. It shouldn't make them. Your experience matters. Your values matter. Your knowledge of your own body matters. These remain central.

Treatment matched to you powered by AI is a powerful tool for your control. It expands your options. It increases precision. It threatens your control when it's presented as inarguable. It threatens your control when it replaces doctor judgment and your preference.

Your AI Health Assistant [NEAR HORIZON]

Within the next few years, you'll likely have access to AI health assistants. They'll connect all aspects of your care. Current technology can't do this yet.

Picture this. A system that connects to all your health data sources. Your medical records. Your fitness tracker. Your symptom journal. Your pharmacy records. Your appointment history. It knows your complete health context. It monitors patterns in real time. It notices when something changes that might be significant.

This AI assistant helps you prepare for appointments. It analyzes your recent symptoms. It suggests relevant questions you might not have thought to ask. It catches potential medication interactions before they happen. It identifies patterns in your data that might show a problem developing. Things that might be invisible when you're looking at individual data points. It translates medical jargon in your test results into plain language. It helps you track what you need to communicate to your care team.

When you have a health decision to make, it pulls together relevant research. It explains trade-offs in clear language. It helps you think through how different options align with your values and priorities. When you're between appointments and something feels wrong, it can help you assess. It determines whether you need urgent care. Or if it can wait.

This isn't science fiction. Pieces of this already exist. Just not connected together yet. Research is actively underway on these connected systems. Studies examine how to combine electronic health records. They combine wearable device data. They combine patient-reported symptoms. They combine all of these into unified AI systems. These provide personalized support.

The evidence on specific applications is concrete. A systematic review of 60 studies published in the Journal of Medical Internet Research found something important. AI combined with wearable devices shows real promise. It helps people with diabetes monitor glucose levels. It helps adjust insulin. It predicts complications before they happen. Other research shows similar potential for heart disease monitoring. Wearable devices and AI work together to catch warning signs early.

The control implications are significant. A good AI health assistant amplifies your capacity. It makes you an informed, prepared, engaged partner in your care. It gives you some of the knowledge and analytical capacity of a medical professional. It supports your role as the central coordinator of your own care.

But patient perspectives reveal important concerns. You need to be aware of these.

A study asked 455 people with chronic conditions what they thought about AI-powered wearable health devices. Most appreciated features like real-time alerts and predictive insights. They also raised concerns. Technical reliability matters. Data accuracy matters. And this is important. Diminished human interaction. People worried that AI systems might replace the human connection. This connection is essential to good care.

Healthcare professionals share similar concerns. Research surveys consistently show that many clinicians express hesitation. They worry about adopting AI systems. They primarily cite concerns. They worry about not understanding how AI makes decisions. They worry about data security.

These concerns matter. As these AI assistant systems roll out, you'll need clarity on important questions and this is where only your doctor can help.

The Doctor-AI Partnership Evolving [AVAILABLE TODAY / EXPANDING]

The relationship between doctors and AI is shifting dramatically. This shift will change your experience of medical care in major ways.

Right now, AI in clinical settings mostly works in the background. Your doctor might use it without you knowing. AI reads your X-rays or CT scans. AI suggests diagnoses to consider. AI flags potential drug interactions.

The doctor remains the primary interface with you.

That's changing. AI is moving from background assistant to active participant. It will be part of your care conversations.

Here's what's starting to happen. Doctors are beginning to use AI during appointments. It supports decision-making in real time. Research from early 2025 examined how 108 physicians around the world used AI help during patient care. They were family doctors, emergency physicians, internists, pediatricians. Another study tested 50 U.S. doctors with AI help for diagnosing chest pain. The results showed that AI improved diagnostic accuracy significantly. It helped doctors catch conditions they might have missed.

In the near future, your appointment might include AI. The AI listens to your conversation with your doctor. It suggests questions neither of you thought to ask. It pulls up relevant research in real-time. It identifies patterns in your symptoms that weren't obvious. The doctor isn't replaced. But the doctor's ability to process information is expanded significantly.

This could be wonderful for your control. Imagine your doctor having instant access to the latest research on your specific condition. Imagine this happening during your appointment. Imagine AI catching a potential dangerous interaction between two of your medications. Imagine this happening before it becomes a problem. Imagine having a "third mind" in the room. That mind brings more perspective without rushing you through your appointment.

The potential upside is significant. More accurate diagnoses. Better matching of treatments to patients. Fewer medical errors. More thorough consideration of options. Doctors who can focus more on the human relationship with you. Why? Because the AI handles the heavy lifting. It handles information retrieval and pattern recognition.

But research also reveals important challenges. AI-based tools have enhanced treatment matched to you. But trust in these tools remains a critical factor. Trust matters for successful adoption. Both patients and doctors must trust the AI for it to work well. And trust has been slow to develop. Partly because doctors don't always understand how the AI reaches its conclusions. Partly because of cultural resistance to change.

There are real risks here too. AI can make doctors overconfident in wrong conclusions. AI can bias thinking toward certain diagnoses. Why? Because of flaws in the information used to teach the AI. AI can become a distraction from actually listening to you. AI can feel like it's making decisions rather than informing them.

The dynamic you want is this. Doctor plus AI working together to serve your needs. You're the central partner in all decisions. A true three-way collaboration where technology enhances rather than replaces human judgment and human connection.

WHAT THIS MEANS FOR YOUR APPOINTMENTS:

You can ask about AI's role. If your doctor is using AI during your appointment, you can say: "I'm curious, how are you using AI in our conversation today?" This isn't confrontational. It's partnership. Most doctors will appreciate your interest.

Many doctors are cautiously optimistic about AI's potential. They also remain appropriately skeptical about its limitations. This is a good thing. They do and will continue to use AI as a tool to enhance their practice of medicine. It won't replace clinical judgment or patient connection, but it can be an additional tool to help them. So don't be afraid when your doctor mentions that he's using AI.

The doctor-AI partnership has enormous potential to improve your care. But it only serves your control when all three partners—you, your doctor, and the AI—are working in transparent collaboration. Your needs must be at the center.

The Human-In-The-Loop Principle

Remember this. The AI is the "third mind" in the room. It can suggest. It can inform. It can support. But only two minds in that room have the authority to make the final call. Yours and your doctor's. The AI's job is to make both of you smarter and more capable. It's a tool, not a decision-maker.

The Equity Questions We Must Ask [ONGOING CONCERN]

Every technology amplifies existing inequalities. Unless we deliberately design it not to. AI in healthcare is no exception.

As these powerful new tools roll out, we have to ask. Who gets access?

Will AI health assistants be available only to people with expensive insurance? Will they only be available to people who can pay out of pocket? Will treatment matched to you powered by AI be a luxury good? Will it widen the gap between those with resources and those without?

Will AI-enabled emotional support reach people in under-resourced communities? Or will it become another benefit that only privileged patients can access?

These aren't abstract questions. They're questions about whether AI makes healthcare more fair or less fair.

Then there's the data problem. This one is serious.

Most medical datasets used to train AI models have historically over-represented certain groups. White patients, people in wealthy countries, patients at major academic medical centers. This means AI models are often better at diagnosing and treating people who look like the patients in the information used to teach the AI.

If you're a woman, a person of color, someone living in a rural area, someone without consistent healthcare access, AI trained on biased information might work less well for you. It might misdiagnose you more often. It might recommend treatments less suitable for your situation. It might miss patterns that are common in your demographic but rare in the information used to teach the AI.

This is already happening. A landmark 2019 study examined a widely used healthcare algorithm. They discovered shocking racial bias. The algorithm was supposed to identify which patients needed extra medical attention. But it systematically rated Black patients as having the same risk level as white patients who were actually much sicker. Because the AI had learned from biased information, it perpetuated and amplified racial inequities in healthcare.

The implications are staggering. Researchers calculated that fixing this bias could help increase the percentage of Black patients receiving necessary more care from 18% to 47%. That's a massive difference in human lives and health outcomes.

A major 2024 review examined racial and ethnic bias in AI health algorithms. They analyzed 23 different sources. The researchers identified six critical themes. AI can perpetuate racial inequities. Fairness should be prioritized in algorithm design. Lack of diversity among AI developers is concerning. Regulation and accuracy testing are needed. Ethical standards must be established. Transparency and accountability are essential.

We're at a critical juncture. Healthcare systems often overlook individual differences. Without deliberate attention to fairness, AI risks amplifying these oversights. AI risks making them worse.

Your Role in Fairness

When AI tools are introduced, you can ask your doctor. "In your experience, does this AI work equally well for patients with different backgrounds?" This is a clinical question your doctor can reflect on. They can reflect on this based on their practice experience.

If you sense something isn't right. "I'm concerned this recommendation doesn't account for [my specific factor]. Can we explore alternatives?" This focuses on your individual case, which is always appropriate.

If you have capacity to share your experience. When AI works well or poorly for you, mentioning it to your care team helps them learn. Your feedback contributes to better outcomes for future patients like you.

You don't have to be a systemic activist to practice fairness-aware control. You just have to be honest about your experience. You have to be persistent in requesting approaches that work for your specific situation.

Privacy in the AI Era [ONGOING CONCERN]

Here's the central trade-off with AI in healthcare. The more AI knows about you, the more helpful it can be. But all of that data needs to be protected.

Your AI health assistant needs access to your medical history. It needs your current symptoms. It needs your treatment responses. Maybe even your genetic information to personalize recommendations. AI companions need to understand your emotional patterns and your specific situation. They need this to provide meaningful support.

But all of that data is intimate. It's valuable. It's potentially vulnerable. As AI systems become more capable, the privacy risks become more complex.

The concerns are real. Research surveys consistently show that many healthcare professionals hesitate to adopt AI systems. Data security and transparency in data use are frequently cited concerns.

The Healthcare System Transformation [HAPPENING NOW]

AI isn't just changing individual tools and conversations. It's transforming the entire healthcare system. It will affect how you access care, what's available to you, and how healthcare pays for itself.

The pace of transformation is remarkable. Remember those numbers from the beginning of this chapter? Doctor AI adoption jumped from 38% to 66% in a single year. Investment capital is flooding into AI healthcare companies. They captured 62% of the 6.4 billion dollars raised by digital health startups in the first half of 2025 alone. This level of investment and adoption suggests the technology is being taken seriously by the healthcare industry. Clinical outcomes continue to be studied and validated.

Some of these changes will make the system more responsive to your needs. Some will create new barriers. You need to understand the landscape that's taking shape.

AI is changing how care gets paid for. Insurance companies increasingly use AI to approve or deny treatment claims. They use AI to predict which patients will be expensive. They use AI to identify what they consider "unnecessary" care. This has serious implications for your access. If an AI determines that your treatment isn't "medically necessary" based on group statistics, you might face denial. This might happen even if you and your doctor believe it's essential for your specific situation.

IF YOUR INSURANCE DENIES CARE BASED ON AI:

You may have specific rights depending on your insurance type and state. Use this script:

INSURANCE APPEAL SCRIPT:

"I'm formally requesting human review of this AI-based denial.

[Note: The right to human review varies by state, insurance type (Medicare/Medicaid/private), and program. Check with your state's insurance commissioner or patient advocate to understand your specific rights.]

I request:

1. The specific criteria the AI used to make this determination
2. Explanation of how these criteria apply to my individual case
3. Review by a licensed medical professional (not an algorithm) who specializes in [your condition]

My physician has recommended this treatment based on my specific clinical presentation. This includes [specific factors the AI may not have considered]. I request reconsideration based on my individual circumstances. Don't use group statistics."

This language asserts your request for human review. Keep a copy of everything you send. If your initial appeal is denied, contact your state's insurance commissioner. You can also contact a patient advocacy organization for guidance on next steps.

AI is changing which providers you can access. Telemedicine powered by AI triage makes it easier to get care from home. This is genuinely helpful for many people. But it also sometimes replaces in-person visits you actually need. It substitutes lower-quality virtual alternatives. An AI system might decide your symptoms can be handled virtually when you really need hands-on examination.

If you believe you need in-person care. "I understand the AI triage suggests virtual care. But I'm requesting an in-person evaluation because [specific reason: I need physical examination, my symptoms require hands-on assessment, virtual visits haven't been effective for this issue]."

AI is changing how appointments work. Some of these changes are positive. AI that handles medical documentation so your doctor can make eye contact with you instead of typing into a computer? That's good. AI that helps schedule appointments more efficiently? Also good.

But some changes are negative. AI-driven productivity metrics push doctors to see more patients in less time. That's bad for you. The appointment feels rushed because it's rushed. The system is measuring doctor "efficiency" in ways that prioritize volume over quality of care.

If your appointments feel rushed. You can say: "I know time is limited, but I need a few more minutes to make sure we've covered everything important. Can we schedule a follow-up if needed?" This acknowledges the reality while advocating for adequate time.

AI is consolidating power. Large healthcare systems and big tech companies can afford to build sophisticated AI tools. Smaller practices can't compete. This reduces your options. It potentially makes care more impersonal.

Understanding these system-level changes helps you navigate more effectively. When you encounter frustrations in your healthcare experience, knowing that institutional pressures might be driving those frustrations helps you respond appropriately. Focus on your individual care while recognizing larger forces at play.

The healthcare system will be different in coming years. AI will largely cause this transformation. That transformation will reflect the priorities we emphasize. As patients request transparency, partnership, and individual consideration, those priorities shape how AI gets deployed.

Your Future, Your Power [YOUR CHOICE ALWAYS]

Let's pull this together. The future of AI in healthcare is arriving fast. Some of what's coming will genuinely help you live better with your condition. You'll make more informed decisions. You'll practice control more effectively. Some of what's coming will threaten to reduce you to data points. It will take power away from you. It will deepen existing inequities.

The question isn't whether AI will transform your healthcare. It will. The question is whether that transformation serves your humanity or diminishes it.

You have more power to influence this than you might think. You're not writing the algorithms. You're not running the tech companies. But you have real power nonetheless.

The power to ask questions. To request transparency. To choose providers who use AI thoughtfully rather than letting it replace judgment. To share what you learn with other patients. To practice control consistently in an AI-enabled world. One appointment. One decision. One conversation at a time.

I want you to remember something as AI becomes more present in your care:

Technology should serve your power, not replace it. Any AI tool that makes you feel less capable, less informed, or less central to decisions about your body deserves questioning. The goal of good healthcare technology is to amplify your capacity. It's not to diminish it.

Convenience isn't the same as care. AI might make some things easier. But if it makes your care less personal, less detailed, or less responsive to your specific needs, that ease comes at too high a cost. Don't trade quality for convenience.

Your experience matters more than the algorithm. AI sees patterns in groups. You aren't a group. You're an individual with specific circumstances. Your lived experience of your body and your condition is irreplaceable data. When there's a conflict between what AI predicts and what you know about your body, your knowledge matters.

Partnership is stronger than skepticism or blind trust. You don't have to embrace every AI tool or reject all of them. You can be thoughtfully selective. Be excited about helpful AI tools while questioning ones that don't serve your needs. This isn't contradictory. It's wise.

You deserve both innovation and humanity. The choice isn't between high-tech care and compassionate care. You can have both. You should have both. AI at its best enhances the human relationship in healthcare. It doesn't replace it.

We're at the beginning of this transformation, not the end. The AI tools available now are primitive compared to what's coming. That's exciting and unsettling in equal measure.

But throughout all the technological change ahead, one thing remains constant. You're a whole person. You're not a collection of data points. You deserve healthcare that sees you, hears you, and partners with you. You deserve to be in control in your pursuit of wellness.

AI can support that control. It can make you more informed, more prepared, more capable of navigating the complex healthcare system. It can give you access to support and information that weren't available to previous generations of patients.

But AI can only support your control if we build it, deploy it, regulate it, and use it with that goal in mind. That requires thoughtfulness. Clear communication with your care team is necessary. Consistent practice of the principles this book has explored is necessary.

The future is coming. You're ready for it. You have the frameworks to evaluate new tools through the lens of control. You have the skills to partner with your healthcare team in an AI-enabled system. You have the understanding of what healthcare should be at its best. Technology-enhanced but fundamentally human.

Keep practicing. Keep questioning. Keep partnering with your care team to ensure your place at the center of your care. No matter how advanced the AI gets, your humanity remains the most important variable in the equation.

THE FINAL WORD: HUMAN-IN-THE-LOOP ALWAYS

As AI becomes more sophisticated, never forget. The algorithm is a tool. Your doctor is a partner. But you're the authority on your own life and body.

AI can suggest. Your doctor can recommend. But you decide.

That's not just control. That's medicine done right. Technology enhances human judgment. It never replaces it.

The journey continues. The technology changes. Your control endures.

You matter more than any algorithm.

Never forget that.

SOURCES

KEY SOURCES (PEER-REVIEWED AND MAJOR MEDICAL ORGANIZATIONS)

AI companions and emotional support

Systematic review and meta-analysis of AI-based conversational agents for promoting mental health and well-being. Nature Digital Medicine. https://www.nature.com/articles/s41746-023-00979-5

Effectiveness of Communication Competence in AI Conversational Agents for Health: Systematic Review and Meta-Analysis.

Journal of Medical Internet Research. https://www.jmir.org/2025/1/e76296

Conversational Agents Supporting Self-Management in People With a Chronic Disease: Systematic Review. Journal of Medical Internet Research. https://www.jmir.org/2025/1/e72309

User perceptions and experiences of an AI-driven conversational agent for mental health support. PMC. https://pmc.ncbi.nlm.nih.gov/articles/PMC11304096/

Charting the evolution of artificial intelligence mental health chatbots from rule-based systems to large language models: a systematic review. PMC. https://pmc.ncbi.nlm.nih.gov/articles/PMC12434366/

PERSONALIZED MEDICINE AND AI

Individualized Medicine in the Era of Artificial Intelligence. Mayo Clinic Proceedings. https://www.mayoclinicproceedings.org/article/S0025-6196(25)00417-3/fulltext

AI-powered precision medicine: utilizing genetic risk factor optimization to revolutionize healthcare. PMC. https://pmc.ncbi.nlm.nih.gov/articles/PMC12051108/

AI health assistants and wearables

Integration of artificial intelligence and wearable technology in the management of diabetes and prediabetes. Nature Digital Medicine. https://www.nature.com/articles/s41746-025-02036-9

Adoption barriers and facilitators of wearable health devices with AI integration: a patient-centred perspective. Frontiers in Medicine. https://www.frontiersin.org/journals/medicine/articles/10.3389/fmed.2025.1557054/full

PHYSICIAN-AI COLLABORATION

Physician clinical decision modification and bias assessment in a randomized controlled trial of AI help. Nature Communications Medicine. https://www.nature.com/articles/s43856-025-00781-2

Trust in Artificial Intelligence–Based Clinical Decision Support Systems Among Health Care Workers: Systematic Review. Journal of Medical Internet Research. https://www.jmir.org/2025/1/e69678

AI-based Clinical Decision Support for Primary Care: A Real-World Study. arXiv preprint (not peer-reviewed). https://arxiv.org/html/2507.16947v1

Healthcare AI bias and equity

Dissecting racial bias in an algorithm used to manage the health of populations. Science (Obermeyer et al., 2019). https://www.science.org/doi/10.1126/science.aax2342

The bias algorithm: how AI in healthcare make worse ethnic and racial disparities: a scoping review. Ethnicity & Health. https://www.tandfonline.com/doi/full/10.1080/13557858.2024.2422848

Bias Mitigation in Primary Health Care Artificial Intelligence Models: Scoping Review. Journal of Medical Internet Research. https://www.jmir.org/2025/1/e60269

Bias recognition and mitigation strategies in artificial intelligence healthcare applications. Nature Digital Medicine. https://www.nature.com/articles/s41746-025-01503-7

PRIVACY AND DATA SECURITY

Balancing Privacy and Progress: A Review of Privacy Challenges, Systemic Oversight, and Patient Perceptions in AI-Driven Healthcare. Applied Sciences. https://www.mdpi.com/2076-3417/14/2/675

The Role of Artificial Intelligence in Safeguarding Patient Privacy in Healthcare Systems. PMC. https://pmc.ncbi.nlm.nih.gov/articles/PMC12244842/

more reading (market context and industry commentary)

How Digital & AI Will Reshape Health Care in 2025. Boston Consulting Group. https://www.bcg.com/publications/2025/digital-ai-solutions-reshape-health-care-2025

Trends 2025: AI in healthcare progressing despite reimbursement hurdles. Healthcare Finance News. https://www.healthcarefinance

news.com/news/trends-2025-ai-healthcare-progressing-despite-reimbursement-hurdles

16

THE FEELING NOBODY
PREPARES YOU FOR

This chapter has nothing to do with AI or checklists or anything other than what it means to be a sovereign patient.

Before we get started, I must remind you I'm writing this as a patient. I am not a doctor, social worker, psychologist, or anything other than a patient living with these realities myself. I don't have it all figured out, and what I share are areas I still struggle with many days.

In many ways, I am writing this chapter to myself. So let's start it that way. Let me stop and get a box of tissues because I have a feeling this might lead to a few tears being shed. OK so let me get started.

And one more thing. If you're in a dark place right now — not just sad, but truly struggling — please put this book down and call or text 988. That's the Suicide and Crisis Lifeline, and they're there for you right now. This chapter will be here when you're ready. Take care of yourself first.

⁓

Dear Dan,

There's a moment that many people with chronic illness know. It is deeply personal. It speaks to your heart.

It doesn't happen during a medical crisis. It doesn't happen at a bad appointment. It happens on an ordinary Tuesday. Or a quiet Sunday morning. Or in the middle of the grocery store.

It's the moment when everything hits you. Not the medical facts — you already know those. Not your treatment plan — you've been following that. It's something deeper. Something harder to name.

It's the emotional reality of your situation. Indefinitely. Without a finish line.

I saw someone my age do something easy. My body no longer allows it. I canceled plans for the third time because my symptoms flared again. Someone said, "You look great!" But that is not how I feel. In fact, I feel anything but great. I smile because explaining the truth would take too much energy.

Nobody prepared me for this part. My doctors talk about symptoms. My pharmacist talks about drug interactions. My insurance company talks about denials. But nobody ever sat me down and said the truth:

This is going to break your heart. You're going to grieve the person you used to be. You'll feel guilty for things that aren't your fault. You'll feel alone even in a room full of people who love you. And all of that is completely normal.

When someone you love dies, the world acknowledges it. People send flowers. They bring food. They give you time and permission to not be okay.

But when you lose your health? When you lose the version of yourself who could work full days? Who could juggle twelve projects? Who could keep up with family conversations without his brain shutting down?

There are no flowers. No ceremony. Nobody sends a card that says, "I'm sorry you lost yourself."

That's what happened to me. After my brain injury, I didn't just lose abilities. I lost the person who had those abilities. I was the marketer who defined himself through what he could produce. That person wasn't coming back. And nobody sent flowers.

This grief doesn't follow neat stages. It comes in waves. I feel okay for weeks, sometimes months. Then a photo from before my diagnosis. Or a conversation about future plans. Or a good day that reminds me of what bad days take away. And it hits all over again.

You will know exactly what I'm talking about. I want you to hear something. This grief isn't weakness. It's not self-pity. It's not a failure to "accept" your condition. It's a completely normal response to real loss. You are allowed to grieve. And at the same time, you can build the best possible life you have. Those two things aren't contradictions.

ＡBOUT EXHAUSTION.

Not the exhaustion of the illness itself. The exhaustion of being a patient.

The medication management. The symptom tracking. The appointment coordination across multiple specialists. The insurance navigation. The prior authorizations. The research. The constant decision-making — is this symptom new or normal? Should I call the doctor or wait? Should I push through today or rest?

Every single day brings dozens of small decisions that healthy people never have to count.

There have been periods when managing my epilepsy felt like a full-time job on top of everything else. Some weeks, the management consumed more energy than the condition itself.

And here's the toughest part: when the work of being a patient gets too big, everything suffers. You can't keep up. So you let something slip. And then you feel guilty. And then the healthcare system labels you "non-compliant." As if you weren't trying hard enough. As if this was a character flaw instead of an impossible workload.

You're not failing at being a patient, Dan. The system is asking too much.

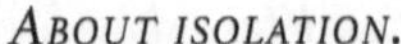

ABOUT ISOLATION.

At the moment when you most need connection, it becomes harder than ever to achieve.

Because you have an invisible condition. You look fine. You're dressed normally. Maybe you're even smiling. So people conclude you must be fine. They don't see the energy it took to get dressed. They don't see the pain behind that smile. They don't see that you'll spend the rest of the day recovering from this one outing.

You can't share the reality of your experience without being seen as complaining. But you can't hide it without feeling increasingly alone. Neither option serves you.

Some surface friendships have drifted away, but some relationships have grown much deeper. But the social landscape shifts underneath you. And the loss of casual, easy connection is another grief nobody acknowledges.

If you feel isolated, I want you to know — it's not because something is wrong with you. It's because the world hasn't built adequate space for your reality. That's not your failure. That's a gap the rest of the world needs to fill.

ABOUT GUILT AND SHAME.

Guilt for not being productive enough. Guilt for needing help. Guilt for being a burden. Guilt for not being "sick enough" on good days. Guilt for being "too sick" on bad days. Guilt for not managing your condition better.

And the performance. The exhausting, daily performance of wellness. Putting on a brave face when you feel anything but a champion. Pushing through social events because canceling again feels too shameful. Answering "I'm doing fine" because explaining the truth would take more energy than you have left.

With epilepsy, there's an extra layer. The fear of having a seizure in public. The fear of being seen as incompetent. Damaged goods. These fears shape daily decisions in ways that few can understand.

ABOUT TOXIC POSITIVITY.

You've heard it all. "Everything happens for a reason." "Just stay positive!" "At least it's not cancer." "You're so strong!" "God only gives you what you can handle." While all of this is true and is usually offered with genuine love. Be careful when these truisms function to shut down what you're actually feeling; when they exist to make the other person more comfortable, they become a kind of dismissal. And you've been dismissed enough.

You don't have to pretend you're okay when you're not. Suppressing what you feel doesn't make it go away. It just drives it underground, where it can get worse. The key is to be honest and realistically optimistic. Be careful not to dwell on the negative or the challenges of the symptoms. This is the real battle. Be positive, but true.

ABOUT GROWTH.

Having been forced down this road, what I've found here matters to me in ways my previous career didn't. My brain injury took away my ability to work the way I used to. That loss was painful and remains painful. The wounds are real and run deep, but the space it created eventually led me to discover a new passion to help others, whether it is through volunteering at the local hospital, taking classes, or seeking out opportunities to help others. That's not a silver lining. It's just what happens when you're human. We build meaning from rubble. Not because the destruction was good. But because meaning-making is what we do.

If you've experienced growth through your illness, don't feel guilty about it. If you haven't, don't feel like you're missing something. Growth isn't an obligation. It's a possibility — one that shows up on its own timeline.

So HERE'S *what I want to say to myself, and to you, in case you need someone to say it:*

Your feelings about being "sick" are valid. The grief, the anger, the exhaustion, the guilt, the fear, the moments of unexpected beauty. All of it. You don't have to justify your emotional experience to anyone. You don't have to perform positivity. You don't have to pretend.

You're not weak for struggling emotionally with something that is, objectively, very hard. You're not failing because you cry sometimes. Or feel nothing at all sometimes. You're responding to a difficult reality with the full range of human emotion. That's not a problem to solve. That's being alive.

And being fully alive — with all the messiness and pain and beauty that implies — is the most sovereign thing you can do.

Your feelings are part of the journey. They always were.

You matter. What you feel matters. Don't let anyone — including yourself — tell you otherwise.

With Love,

If this chapter surfaced feelings you need help processing, you're not alone, and support is available: 988 Suicide and Crisis Lifeline (call or text 988, available 24/7) or Crisis Text Line (text HOME to 741741). For help finding a therapist, visit psychologytoday.com. You deserve professional support — asking for it is sovereignty in action.

ACKNOWLEDGMENTS

This book exists because I had help when I needed it most.

To my wife: You saw me when the medical system didn't. When doctors called me a "challenging patient," you called me resilient. When I couldn't find the words through brain fog, you helped me organize my thoughts. When I wanted to give up on being heard, you reminded me that my voice mattered. This book is as much yours as mine.

To the Mayo Clinic teams who listened: Thank you for treating me as a partner, not a problem. Your willingness to work collaboratively gave me a model for what patient-centered care could look like.

To Dr. Freund: You were the first doctor to ask "What's it like?" instead of just "What are the symptoms?" That question changed everything. It showed me that genuine curiosity about patient experience is possible in medicine.

To the online chronic illness community: Your stories, your frameworks (yes, Spoon Theory), and your willingness to share both struggles and strategies gave me language for experiences I thought were mine alone. You taught me that being a challenging patient is often a sign of having a challenging condition, not a personal failing.

To every patient who has shared their story with me: Your experiences shaped this book. Your frustrations validated mine. Your victories gave me hope. Every framework in these pages was tested and refined through conversations with people navigating their own healthcare journeys.

To the AI researchers and healthcare technologists working to build tools that empower rather than extract: Your work gives me optimism about what's possible. Special thanks to those who prioritize transparency, patient access, and equity in medical AI.

To my former clients and colleagues in the marketing world: The skills you helped me develop—asking better questions, organizing complex information, challenging assumptions—turned out to be exactly what I needed as a patient. That career wasn't a detour from this work; it was preparation for it.

To healthcare providers who are trying to practice differently despite systemic constraints: I see you. I know the system makes true partnership difficult. This book critiques structures, not people. Thank you for the moments of genuine connection that happen despite the barriers.

To everyone living with chronic illness: You are the reason this book exists. Your expertise about your own body is real, valuable, and irreplaceable. You deserve to be seen, heard, and treated as the sovereign expert on your own experience.

And finally, to my brain: We've had a complicated relationship since the injuries and seizures began. You've betrayed me, frustrated me, and humbled me. But you've also taught me things I couldn't have learned any other way. We're learning to coexist. Thank you for the unexpected education.

This book was written through brain fog, between seizures, during the moments when clarity returned. If it helps even one person feel less alone in their healthcare journey, every difficult word was worth it.

RESOURCES

Additional Reading and References

The following resources can support your journey toward healthcare sovereignty. This list represents a starting point—not an endorsement of every claim or approach, but a collection of tools and organizations that may be helpful as you navigate chronic illness and advocate for your care.

Organizations & Advocacy Groups

Patient Advocacy Organizations - Patient Advocate Foundation (patientadvocate.org) - Free case management for chronic illness patients - National Patient Advocate Foundation (npaf.org) - Policy advocacy and healthcare access - Center for Patient Partnerships (law.wisc.edu/patientadvocacy) - Patient-centered advocacy training

    Chronic Illness Support - Chronic Illness Advocacy & Awareness Network (chronicillnessaa.org) - The Mighty (themighty.com) - Stories and community for chronic illness - Spoon Theory Community (butyoudontlooksick.com) - Understanding energy management

Healthcare Rights & Navigation - Patient Rights Advocate (patientrightsadvocate.org) - Transparency in healthcare pricing - Healthcare Advocates (healthcareadvocates.com) - Professional healthcare navigation - Patient Family & Consumer Center at Johns Hopkins (patient.hopkinsmedicine.org) - Patient-centered resources

Books on Patient Advocacy & Healthcare

Understanding the Healthcare System - *Being Mortal* by Atul Gawande - How medicine shapes end-of-life care - *The Patient Will See You Now* by Eric Topol - Digital transformation of healthcare - *An American Sickness* by Elisabeth Rosenthal - How healthcare became big business

Chronic Illness & Patient Experience - *The Body Keeps the Score* by Bessel van der Kolk - Trauma and healing - *When Breath Becomes Air* by Paul Kalanithi - A doctor becomes a patient - *How to Be a Patient* by Sana Goldberg - Practical guide to medical care - *In Shock* by Rana Awdish - A doctor's journey through serious illness

Medical Decision-Making - *Your Medical Mind* by Jerome Groopman and Pamela Hartzband - Making medical choices - *The Checklist Manifesto* by Atul Gawande - Systems thinking for safety - *Overdiagnosed* by H. Gilbert Welch - Understanding medical testing

AI & Technology in Healthcare

Understanding Medical AI - FDA's AI/ML-Enabled Medical Devices List (fda.gov/medical-devices) - Current approved AI tools - Healthcare Information and Management Systems Society (HIMSS) (himss.org) - Health IT standards - AI for Healthcare (ai4healthcare.org) - Education on medical AI

Health Data & Privacy - HealthIT.gov - Official government health IT resource - MyHealthEData (healthit.gov/topic/health-it-initiatives/myhealthedata) - Patient access to medical records - Health Insurance Portability and Accountability Act Resource Center (hhs.gov/hipaa) - Understanding privacy rights

Practical Tools & Apps

Health Tracking & Organization - Apple Health, Google Fit - Basic health tracking - MyChart, Epic - Hospital-based patient portals - Medisafe, MyTherapy - Medication management - PatientsLikeMe - Health tracking and community

    Mental Health Support - Woebot, Wysa - AI-powered mental health support - BetterHelp, Talkspace - Online therapy platforms - NAMI (nami.org) - Mental health education and support

    Medical Research - PubMed (pubmed.ncbi.nlm.nih.gov) - Free access to medical research - ClinicalTrials.gov - Information on clinical studies - Cochrane Library (cochranelibrary.com) - Systematic reviews of medical research

Support for Specific Conditions

Given the diversity of chronic conditions, I recommend searching for condition-specific organizations through: - National Organization for Rare Disorders (RARECARE.org) - American Chronic Pain Association (theacpa.org) - National Alliance on Mental Illness (nami.org) - Condition-specific foundations (American Heart Association, Epilepsy Foundation, etc.)

Downloadable Tools

Visit [website URL] for free downloadable versions of the frameworks in this book: - Health Dashboard Template - Appointment Preparation Checklist - Question Card - Six Elements of Transformative Conversations - Insurance Appeal Template - Three AM Practice - Self-Compassion Reset

NOTES ON SOURCES

Rather than interrupt the narrative flow with numbered citations, I've chosen to acknowledge key research and sources that informed this book. This approach honors both readability and intellectual honesty.

Chapter-by-Chapter Research Foundation

Chapter 3: The Hidden AI Already in Your Care The discussion of algorithmic decision-making in healthcare draws on work by Obermeyer et al. (2019) on racial bias in healthcare algorithms, published in *Science*. The FDA's evolving regulatory framework for AI/ML medical devices shaped my understanding of current AI deployment.

Chapter 6: What AI Can and Can't See Research on AI limitations in medical diagnosis comes from multiple sources, including work by Topol (2019) on deep medicine and systematic reviews of AI diagnostic accuracy. The discussion of algorithmic bias draws on Rajkomar et al. (2018) published in *NEJM*.

Chapter 11: Transformative Conversations The framework for shared decision-making builds on decades of research by Elwyn, Frosch, and others. Motivational interviewing principles come from Miller and Rollnick's foundational work.

Chapter 13: The Healthcare You Deserve The critique of the extraction paradigm synthesizes work by multiple healthcare economists and system analysts, including work on fee-for-service limitations and patient-centered care models.

Chapter 15: What's Coming Statistics on FDA-approved personalized medicines and AI diagnostic tools come from FDA databases and industry reports current as of 2025. Research on AI emotional support apps includes studies of Woebot and similar platforms published in peer-reviewed journals.

Chapter 16: The Feeling Nobody Prepares You For The discussion of grief in chronic illness draws on Charmaz (1983) and Eakes, Burke, and Hainsworth (1998) on chronic sorrow. Research on emotional suppression versus acceptance comes from Hayes and colleagues' work on Acceptance and Commitment Therapy. The discussion of Post-Traumatic Growth references Tedeschi and Calhoun's framework.

Full citations and additional reading recommendations are available at dannoyes.com/S2S

ABOUT THE AUTHOR

You might wonder why a marketing communications guy is writing about healthcare AI. Fair question.

Dan Noyes spent 25 years helping Fortune 1000 brands communicate clearly. Then a series of brain injuries led to epilepsy, and he found himself on the other side of communication — trying to be heard by a healthcare system that wasn't always listening.

That experience lit a fire. Dan earned over 40 certifications in healthcare AI from Stanford, Johns Hopkins, Wharton, Google, and other institutions. Not because he wanted a new career, but because he needed to understand the tools that were changing his care. He is a Health Union Certified Patient Leader who writes from the intersection of strategic expertise and daily lived experience with chronic illness.

This is his first book. He lives with his wife and still manages his epilepsy every day. Some days are better than others. All of them are sovereign.

For updates, resources, and community, visit https://dannoyes.com/sovereign-patient or email dan@dannoyes.com.